27 Days in November
Daisy's Story

Sue Hodlin

Published by New Generation Publishing in 2022

Copyright © Sue Hodlin 2021

First Edition

The author asserts the moral right under the Copyright, Designs and Patents Act 1988 to be identified as the author of this work.

All Rights reserved. No part of this publication may be reproduced, stored in a retrieval system or transmitted, in any form or by any means without the prior consent of the author, nor be otherwise circulated in any form of binding or cover other than that which it is published and without a similar condition being imposed on the subsequent purchaser.

ISBN   978-1-80369-207-4

www.newgeneration-publishing.com

New Generation Publishing

Dedication: I wrote this story for Daisy, and for Sam, who had to unknowingly endure too much and keeps me going, for Sue, and the girls, Ava and Amelia, Daisy's nieces, to tell them about Daisy. I wish Tim could read it.

I wrote this for Jan, Daisy's aunt, consistently caring, and for Cherry and Michael, always there for Daisy.

I wrote this book for Daisy, and for everyone who has known and who knows Daisy, and for all those who will come to know her.

Contents

Chapter One: What Happened First 3

Chapter Two: Early Days 13

Chapter Three: An Accident....................................17

Chapter Four: Independent Years............................26

Chapter Five: Memories for Daisy 33

Chapter Six: The Deepening Crisis 49

Chapter Seven: Early Days in Tehran 60

Chapter Eight: 23 November 1996...........................67

Chapter Nine: London 1974 78

Chapter Ten: Daisyness..90

Chapter Eleven: Waking Up....................................94

Chapter Twelve: On the Road 97

Chapter Thirteen: Sunshine 102

Chapter Fourteen: The End Nears 112

Chapter Fifteen: A World That Went to Pieces 118

Chapter Sixteen: A Lucky Escape..........................121

Chapter Seventeen: Traveller's Tales.....................130

Chapter Eighteen: The World is Changing 136

Chapter Nineteen: A World Falls Apart.................140

Appendix 154

Acknowledgements 157

Endnotes 158

Everyone has a story to tell and can usually tell it themselves, but I can't tell you my story so my mum, Sue, is going to tell it for me.

I can tell you my name - it's Daisy.

This is Daisy's story, of what happened to our daughter Daisy. It is a story of illness, of treatment, of recovery, of collapse, of the aftermath. It is an attempt to answer the question - what did happen to Daisy? And it is a tribute to Daisy, the survivor.

Órgiva, Andalusia, Spain

On a dusty patch of ground at the edge of a small mountain village in southern Spain, a group of friends gather on a warm Sunday for a game of boules. The boules are old and scratched. The group of friends is mixed: me, a 'half' resident in Spain, out for the summer months, Oss, a sculptor and engineer who retreated to Spain many years ago but regularly makes forays back to the UK, plunging in a tiny claustrophobic submarine into the cold grey North Sea to service the giant oil rigs above, two young locals from the village and a retired teacher now running a literary retreat in the hills. Oss, a great friend, rolls his silver boule in a good straight line towards the jack. On the way it hits a rogue rock, rolls, stops, rolls again down and away into the dry earth until it bumps to rest against an almond tree. Oss shrugs. His team of three is now losing.

"It's such moments that change life," he jokes.

Out of nowhere, sharp hot tears press my eyes. Picture slides run in my head; the moment Daisy was born, the unbelievable joy of her brother Sam's birth, Daisy as a small child, turning onto her stomach for the very last scan of the back of the head, where, finally, the tumour showed. Nothing seems unusual to us. The technician in the consulting room handing over to us the rolled-up scan.

"I'm so sorry," he said. We were slightly puzzled. Why, we thought? Why was he so sorry?

Daisy remembers how she used to potter about, sweeping up the leaves in the garden, dead heading the roses, but now, confined to a wheelchair, sitting outside at our home in the early Spanish sun, she greets the morning, "Hello world!" with no sentiment, no regret, no bitterness, no sadness of a life past and what has happened to her.

Chapter One

What Happened First

IRAN 1974
Tehran, 17/04/74

To whom it may concern
This is to certify that Daisy Hodlin, a two and a half-year-old girl, has been referred to me with a history of vomitings of ten days' duration. There was also a suggestion of ataxic gait[i]. Her neurological examination revealed no positive finding save for ataxia.

Then, an almost casual sentence that changes everything.

X-rays of the skull and brain scans confirmed the presence of a lesion in the brain, most likely a tumour. It is advisable to take her to England for further care.

K. Abbasioun M.D.
Neurosurgeon.

We had been living in Iran for nearly three years. An exciting, exotic place to be. Iran then was then pre-Revolution. The Shah ruled. A country aspiring to be...who knows? My husband Tim was working in British Council offices in Tehran while I looked after our new baby, Daisy, and later Sam, her brother. I hoped to carry on with my English language teaching and research.

We had never been to Iran, so, before setting off, both of us were given the chance to begin to learn Farsi. Tim had completed a Masters in South East Asian studies, part of which required him to study the Thai language. We had previously lived in Thailand. For months before his final language exam, our flat had been littered with little cut out pieces of card, each with a Thai word written on one side, and the English translation on the other. To no avail. In his exam, seeing the word "cancer", and understanding little else, Tim concocted a translation into English about the treatment of cancer in Thai hospitals. The passage turned out to be about the spread of communism "like a cancer" in South East Asia. Both of us had previously managed to learn and speak some market Thai as graduate volunteers posted to a northern Thai university. Before that, immediately after finishing A levels at school, I had worked in Thailand with Voluntary Service Overseas (VSO), as an assistant at a government girls' secondary.

Farsi was just as difficult as Thai, and our teacher, Ahmad B, could never allow Tim to get more marks than me. Ahmad and his brothers became our friends, and still are to this day.

Within two days of Dr Abbasioun's letter, three of us, Daisy, our eight-month-old Sam and I, leave Iran suddenly and immediately. Tim stays behind to continue at work as we anticipate an early return after an operation to remove Daisy's tumour. But I was not to go back and would not return at all until twenty years later. In 1974, I left with only the jeans and a tee -shirt I was wearing, taking nothing much with me, thinking, this will soon be over, Daisy will have an operation and we will be back. Although medical equipment in Tehran at that time was good, (the type of scanner used was not in common use in the UK), all nursing care fell to relatives, and we thought that might be risky. At first, I was going to leave Sam behind in Tehran to be looked after by friends but, at the very last minute, I felt I needed to take him with me.

On the hastily booked flight back to the UK, the three of us have been allocated only one seat. Me, two-year-old Daisy and baby Sam. Somewhere up in the skies, Daisy projectile vomits once again. When order is restored, we find we now have the whole row to ourselves. At Heathrow Airport, we have the strange embarrassment of an ambulance waiting for us on the tarmac. I am not ill, Sam is asleep, and Daisy looks and behaves like a jolly two-year-old. The ambulance takes us straight to St Bartholomew's Hospital in London. A diversion is made en route to leave Sam with a close relative. How strange, Sam is dropped off as if on a play date. It's now deep nighttime. On arrival at St Bart's, Daisy is put in a big bed and looks very pretty in a soft hospital gown patterned with pink rosebuds. I have no idea where I slept that night, and just remember standing, cold, at pay phones in dark corridors, relaying through an operator what was happening to Tim, who was still in Iran. As events unfold and an operation becomes the obvious next step, rapid plans are made for Tim to return as soon as he can.

Before our trip to the hospital in Tehran, Daisy is healthy a two-year-old. She hasn't been ill at all, but suddenly, one day, she is sick. Then, daily but irregularly, there is unexpected projectile vomiting.

This kind of vomiting is alarming, as if a button has been pressed hard. It's not dribbling stop start sick, just a straight out, strong stream. These streams even become a little bit normal to us. We take a bowl and towel with us in the car each time we go out along with other baby and toddler stuff. Quick checks are made at the doctors. No, it's definitely not her stomach. Next, a quick x-ray – no, thank goodness, it's not a hidden fractured skull. Quick blood test – no, it's not an allergy, and it's not an infection. So, we progress to a scan.

In Iran, such investigations happen quickly. The Mayo Clinic educated doctors correctly identify a medullablastoma, a brain stem tumour. We pay twenty-five tomans (in 1974 about £2.50p) and take the long rolled up paper sheet of the scan the technician hands us home.

"I'm so sorry," he says. Those gentle words repeat in our heads.

That evening, we phone our friend (Dr) Anthony Hopkins[ii], a doctor and a neurologist. We carefully spell out what is written, what is suspected, and what is faintly typed, at the bottom of the scan report sheet.

"Why do all my friends always think their children have brain tumours?" Anthony says to his wife.

In an extraordinary twist of fate, Anthony is the Consultant Neurologist at St Bartholomew's Hospital when Daisy is to be admitted. Years ago, as students, Tim and I had watched some neurological experiments in his lab in troubled, fascinated astonishment, as one of the monkeys in the trial bit Anthony. Now we are in that "unfortunate group of families" of patients with malignant brain tumours.

ST BARTHOLOMEW'S HOSPITAL, SMITHFIELD SQUARE, LONDON
APRIL 24, 1974

Mr. Currie, Daisy's neurosurgeon, spends the whole morning studying and planning the operation. At the time, this seems very strange but very reassuring to us. Before the operation is agreed, Tim and I have an argument at Daisy's bedside as to whether to go ahead with an operation at all, and with the fierce treatment that would follow, while Mr. Currie stands quietly by. Why, if she is going to die, I argue, should she have her last moments in pain, and in hospital? But Tim triumphs. Of course, we must take the chance for her.

I have no memory at all of the last sight we had of Daisy on the morning of the operation, despite trying, really trying, to remember. I still can't remember, even now. As we will have to wait a long time, we leave hospital and spend hour after hour walking round and round in calm Kew Gardens near where Tim's family live, carrying little Sam with us, staring at plants, gazing at pictures in the Marianne North Gallery. Then, leaving Sam behind with Tim's sister again, we drive back to the hospital along that route that will become so familiar. Onto the West Way, up onto the flyover, crawling in traffic jams past Euston Station and St Paul's, finally arriving at Bart's, parking on the curved green opposite the entrance. These are blank memories; the deep and frozen fear and pain of that time stay buried still.

And there she is, there is Daisy, now in a bigger adult bed, paler, tinier, very still, a crinkly, cream crepe bandage like a broad headband on her head, her eyes closed, her long dark lashes against her small, smooth cheeks, perfect.

med * ul * lo * blas * to * ma   medulloblastoma or medullablastoma
Noun, anatomy.
medulla (the hindmost part of the brain) + blastoma (germ) + oma (tumour)
A brain tumour composed of medullablasts. A tumour consisting of neoplastic cells that resemble the undifferentiated cells of the primitive medullary tube; medullablastomas are usually located in the vermis of the cerebellum, brainstem, and spinal cord; they comprise approximately 3% of all intracranial neoplasms, and occur most frequently in children; the neoplastic cells are compactly arranged, rounded or ovoid, with hyperchromatic nuclei and relatively scant cytoplasm, and lie in small and poorly defined groups, or, occasionally, in a pseudo rosette pattern.
A type of neuroectodermal tumour.
Farlex Partner Medical Dictionary 2012[iii]

Medullablastomas are extremely radiosensitive and grow rapidly.
The prognosis is poor.
Mosby's Medical Dictionary 2009[iv]

Mortality
Infants: This group is defined as patients younger than 3 years. (Daisy is 2 years, 7 months and 16 days old). This group has the worst prognosis. The 5-year survival rate is approximately 30%.

Despite successful treatment, a significant number of patients have neurocognitive and endocrinology deficits.
Tobey J MacDonald MD[v]

The prognosis is poor, the 5-year survival rate is 30%. Unbelievable. Writing this now, it is the first time that I have looked at these definitions. Tim and I were being overwhelmed by what was happening to Daisy, but we weren't being overwhelmed by information. In those days, time sped along. A new baby, a move to living abroad, a second baby, a full and interesting life lived day-to-day. No Google, no mobile phones, no internet; we had no way of making further investigations about Daisy's illness. It was just, relentlessly, insidiously, happening.

Daisy arrives back in a ward after an operation seven hours long, almost a whole day. There is a plastic tap with a tube that drains liquid from her head. She is still, puffy, small.

Mr. Currie comes to brief us. He is excited, pleased.

"I got it all out. It was this size." His hands cup in the shape of a tangerine.

Removing as much tumour as possible is an important step in treating medullablastoma. The neurosurgeon has three goals for the surgery: to relieve cerebrospinal fluid buildup caused by the tumour or swelling; to confirm the diagnosis by obtaining a tissue sample, and to remove as much tumour as possible while causing minimal, or no, neurological damage. Several studies have shown that the best chance for long-term tumour control is when all of the medullablastoma visible to the neurosurgeon's eye is safely removed.
American Brain Tumor Association[vi]

Mr. Currie's reliable eye. He got it all out.

ST BARTHOLOMEW'S HOSPITAL, SMITHFIELD SQUARE, LONDON
APRIL 1974

After the removal of her brain tumour, Daisy is placed back in a small, adult ward. She is not placed in Intensive Care and she is not in a children's ward. We don't feel afraid. It amuses us, as we sit by her bed, to listen to the routine neurological tests being done on the old man in the next bed.

Doctor: "Can you tell me what year it is?"
Patient: (pauses) "1974." (It was.)
Doctor: "And can you tell me who the Prime Minister is?"
Patient: Silence. His eyes are closed. A resigned sigh.

Maybe there is a better question to ask. But the old man has his way any way, refusing attempts to complete the questions or accept the offers of food; he just makes himself clear with "no more, no more".

Yes, no more of any of this.

In that side ward at the end of a corridor, somewhere in the hospital, Daisy is being monitored after the operation. There are just four beds. Daisy is in the bed directly opposite the nurses' station on the other side of the half glass wall. The old man is in the bed by the window. A sleeping shape is in another bed. One bed is empty. The room is warm. Daisy is only wearing her nappy. A white terry towelling nappy, a small smooth child's chest, a clean, white-bandaged head. It doesn't look as if her hair has been cut off, but it has. At the bottom of the bed is a white un-creased sheet, folded over. Daisy is on her back, lying quite straight with one leg bent out uncovered. It's quite hot still and quite late at night.

Everyone breathes with their new baby, watches each breath taken, in and out, immediately anxious if their baby sleeps too long or too little. And now we are taking every breath with her again, in rhythm with the slight movement as her chest rises and falls. You can see her ribs. Daisy is motionless. Only her ribs are moving. In and out, slower, in -, and out, in -, and out. Then, there seems to be a strange reverse movement. Her small chest hollows backwards and caves in slightly. Tim is sitting on a chair squashed in behind the bed, absorbed in reading; I am sitting at the side of the bed, fixedly watching. It doesn't look quite right. I look at that flat chest and the slow-motion breath.

I have often wondered, why did I hesitate at that moment? Stay calm under pressure, when there is such a fine, fine line between panic and calm, between living and dying.

Once, as graduate volunteers in northern Thailand, Tim and I went *bei tio*, on a fun day out. We went to the river for a picnic. The wide, muddy river water looked invitingly cool. Tim, who was a good strong swimmer, dived in. I, who was not, stayed on the bridge. I was lost in thought, but, after a while, I looked up and saw Tim, bobbing, far, far away down the river. Too far to see, as I know now, his waving arm, the panic on his face, the splashing. He got out of the river and walked shakily back. A fierce current had seized him and dragged him, helpless, under the water, way downstream. A lucky escape. Stay calm.

Now in that quiet ward, somewhere in that huge hospital, I stand up and cautiously approach the nurse who quietly sits writing at her desk, which is spread with notes, to explain. She walks in to look. Then everything speeds up. She runs out. It is the middle of the night, but Daisy is suddenly surrounded. It's very crowded now round her tiny figure in the bed. The on-duty night registrar is running down the corridor, his white coat flung on, open, over pyjamas. He picks up the oxygen mask at the foot of Daisy's bed and swears. It's far too big for her face. The nurse runs back to her station and grabs a stapler from her desk. She clips the mask smaller to fit tightly over Daisy's white-parchment pale face. Leaning pressed against the wall, I look at the clock outside. 7.15am. Born at 7.15 am in Queen Charlotte's, Chiswick, delivered by Nurse Greenwood in her neat purple uniform and matching purple eye shadow, and now, two years and eight months later, surrounded by nurses and doctors bent over her, Daisy is about to die, at 7.15am, in St Bartholomew's, London.

On a yellowing tiny page torn from a little notepad Tim has scribbled in desperately deteriorating writing:

malignant
tumour
more chance malignant
x-ray
surgery 6 weeks
good chance
2 months

Chapter Two

Early Days

QUEEN CHARLOTTE'S HOSPITAL,
HAMMERSMITH, LONDON
SEPTEMBER 8, 1971. 7.15 AM

Daisy was born so quickly that, although we had borrowed Tim's dad's car to drive to hospital early in the morning, we were able to return it to him before he left for work. No time for painkillers for me. No time to take off my jewellery; I couldn't understand why my shaking hand could not unclasp the bracelet on my wrist, so it stayed on, half-clasped. No time to recite my chosen poem, 'MacCavity The Mystery Cat', as instructed at those National Childbirth Trust Classes. (I hadn't ever learned it properly anyway, so I was quite relieved.)

Daisy Amabelle Hodlin. Tim and I had been reading Scott Fitzgerald's *The Great Gatsby* with its heroine, Daisy Buchanan. Daisy would be the name. Amabel (as it really should be spelt) was a great aunt on the Hodlin side of the family. Daisy isn't sure about her name. Once, in a busy supermarket I called to her, "Daisy!" and she responded, "Don't call me Daisy".

"Well, what shall I call you?"

A pause. "Darling".

I tried to explain I couldn't walk round a supermarket calling "Darling!" (Now, Daisy gets a few other names from me: Little Dorrit, Margarita (in Spain), Ashopan, the eagle huntress of Kazakhstan, Daisybelle and Bella...)

Daisy was a very satisfactory, compact baby. A Virgo. Small and neat, with Hodlin knees. 3.02 kilos, 49 centimetres long, circumference of head 34.5 centimetres. A head that was to be cut, bruised, stitched, radiated, filled with chemicals. Dark blue eyes, brown hair which quickly turned into fairer curls. Daisy had her first hair cut at the Hilton Hotel in Tehran. In April 1974, these fair little curly strands, will be cut off and given to us to keep. They still lie, flattened in an old yellowing envelope, which has scribbled on it, *Daisy's hair*.

We left hospital early after her birth, Daisy and me, before the lesson learning about how to put on a nappy. In those days before disposable nappies, back at home, I thumbed through Dr Spock's *Baby and Child Care* to try and find out about how it should be done, how to grasp and fold the tough towelling and push the blunt nappy pin through the thick, coarse cloth. I don't remember any other books being available to consult then, nor, of course, was the internet available. A friend explained where to put those new mysterious things, nappy liners (it turned out to be inside the terry towelling nappy, of course).

Daisy was not willing to feed to any schedule as instructed in hospital in those days (a true indication of her character). I was determined to breastfeed her. In those early days at home, our joint obstinacy already established. Tim had hired a TV to watch -what? I can't remember, but it was clearly more interesting than watching those (theoretically) 4-hourly feeds. (We never, ever managed to last that full, magic 4 hours.)

ST. BARTHOLOMEW'S HOSPITAL, SMITHFIELD
SQUARE, LONDON
APRIL TO AUGUST 1974.

No breakfast and no lunch is allowed for Daisy who
has to have a general anaesthetic before the daily
radiotherapy treatment that follows her operation. So,
the hospital lunchtime smells are avoided with walks
outside, whatever the weather, as we push her through
Smithfield Market (I learn all about mutton), round the
old walls of the Barbican and along the embankment
by the grey, threatening, swirling River Thames.
Daisy, little and hunched, slightly covered in an old,
colourless, stiff rain cape found by the hospital,
wearing tiny, borrowed slippers, pale bare legs, sitting
in an outdated, dull green, upright hospital pushchair.
The grey, twilight grey, brown grey, watery deep River
Thames.

Frightening (to us) procedures become routine. There are
lumbar punctures frequently to obtain cerebrospinal fluid
(CSF) to measure pressure and to look for chemicals that
may affect brain function. We accompany Daisy each
time and hold her back steady and still so the needle can
be inserted. Our large adult hands span across her small
back, and we can't look away. Is this why I can't now
look at any injection, and why I have to breathe deeply to
give Daisy daily insulin injections? Given the chance, I
shut my eyes at anything like this. Daisy and I both spent
years watching *Casualty* on TV through peeping fingers.

Lumbar puncture procedure.
Your child lies on their side and is held still, with their
knees tucked into their chest and head bent forward.

Babies will be curled in a ball. Young children will be held in this position by an assistant (that's us). A doctor puts a needle between the bones of the lower back. It's an uncomfortable and sometimes painful test. Your child will be held still, and small children do not like this and will often cry[1]. A small number of children may have a headache or back ache for a day or two after the test.

The Royal Children's Hospital General Medicine and Emergency Medicine, Melbourne, Australia. Kidsinfo fact sheet. First published December 2003 (thirty years too late for us.)

Today, our GP friend reflects on the preparation we had for the treatment of Daisy's tumour. (None). Now, she explains, we would have had a cancer nurse with us from the moment of diagnosis, and we would have been given a huge amount of information. Treatment and consultations would be recorded on our smartphones and websites signposted. Patients create blogs (blogs?) and seek out blogs so to be much better informed about diagnosis and to quickly develop virtual support networks across the world. But how much information could we have processed? Were we told the statistics for survival? (No). They were pretty grim at that stage. Medullablastomas were only first diagnosed in 1925 (Bailey and Cushing), when they were uniformly fatal.

---

[1] Now I remember, suddenly. This was one of the few occasions during these months that Daisy did cry, abruptly, distressingly. And headaches? Probably, of course, but who knows what a headache is like for a two-year-old? The tests took place relentlessly often.

Chapter Three

An Accident

THE FARM, WEST MOORS, DORSET.
NOVEMBER 22, 1996.
DAISY IS 25.
DAY 1.
THE MORNING.

After her school years and college, at last some longer lasting calm comes in to our lives when Daisy moves to Sturts Farm, a Camphill farm community in Dorset. *A Place Where Everyone Grows*. In this Community Farm, there are ninety acres of space: arable land, woodland, a market garden and nursery, greenhouses, orchards, beautiful clean animals.

In the 1990s, this particular farm, in the popular New Forest area in the south west of the UK, is quickly being surrounded by expanding villages and estates of new, smart commuter houses. This growing population seeks quicker routes to get to work and to shop. The planners plan a new road straight through and across the farm - they had plenty of space, didn't they? This is the new road proposal, retrieved from a dull looking flyer.

West Moors By-Pass

- The B3027 Station Road through the centre of West Moors is generally below standard.
- The road has a poor accident record.
- Noise, pollution, vibration, danger and delays make conditions unpleasant for those living, working or shopping in West Moors.

What are your views?
Route Y
Route R
Route G
Route B
Do nothing

Talkative and strangely articulate farm companion Daisy (being the shy retiring type she is...), is chosen to speak against the proposal on behalf of the farm community during a three-minute local TV slot. We are asked, and give our permission, for Daisy to take part.

The seven strong (as it was in those days) film crew from the local TV station assemble to put together the piece. They come on a sunny day, look around and select one of the farm's peaceful fields in which to film. They choose to feature Henry, a handsome, big brown and white carthorse, son of Guinevere, one of the farm's many animals. Henry, with his huge, fluffy hooves. Daisy is to say her bit while holding Henry's thick brown leather halter. Filming goes on all day.

Daisy does her stuff and speaks up vociferously and coherently against the plans. Good job, Daisy.

No one really knows what happens next. Maybe the sun glints on the camera in the far hedge and caught Henry's soft brown eye. Maybe Henry is just bored after long hours of standing still, and this is why, on that day in November, Henry suddenly rears up and sets off at a gallop. Daisy, still holding his halter, does not let go and so is jerked and dragged, slithering down to the ground. Henry clatters up… and down, up… and down, up… and down…moving fast across the field. Daisy is still holding on. The cameraman later tells us he heard bones snap as Henry cantered on, oblivious. Down comes his huge hoof, hard bone fringed with silky flying hair, onto Daisy's small leg in its plum-coloured corduroy trouser.

We learnt later that the producer had asked to be allowed to shoot some additional footage of Daisy, probably because before the shoot Daisy had been stroking and talking to two horses in the field and seemed to be comfortable doing this. The proposed road was never started.

Tim, a journalist himself, knows how it works. In a letter to the television company, howling with pain, Tim writes:

…having completed an interview with the team, she was asked to hold the halter of a young, unbroken and (according to the producer) 'frisky' carthorse for an establishing shot. The horse bolted, dragging Daisy under its back hooves, breaking her left leg in two places. Y (the producer) informed me that Daisy 'had told him of her experience with horses" and so he felt it was all right to ask her to hold the animal.

Daisy is 4' 8", (she still is) the carthorse some 16 hands. A cute shot. While she has been trained with riding horses, she has never worked with unbroken carthorses. It is rather like throwing someone into a cage of tigers having been told they are experienced with domestic cats.

Daisy had indeed been trained with riding horses. Leaving behind the bumpy road of school, aged just sixteen, she went to a special centre in the New Forest where life skills were taught through horsemanship. Daisy was soon able to ride horses almost like an acrobat, in the light blue tailored blouse and tie and dark blue jodhpurs uniform of the centre, arms held outstretched wide, round and rhythmically round the paddock arena.

POOLE HOSPITAL, DORSET, SOUTH WEST ENGLAND
NOVEMBER 22, 1996.
DAY 1
EARLY AFTERNOON.

Tim, at home in Brighton, speaks to Daisy on a phone held to her ear in the ambulance as it waits at the entrance to Poole Hospital. Tim sends a message to me at work. I am in the middle of a weekly staff meeting, but a really special one as it is the final discussion of our preparations for the government inspection beginning next week where success will propel the education centre where I work into essential authorized and quality recognized status. Daisy is pretty excited, but cross too because the paramedics have cut off her favourite plum red, corduroy trousers. We imagine she will be very pleased to have for once a visible disability, a nice big, plastered leg ready for everyone to sign and draw on. When we arrive at the hospital two hours or so later, we find she is still waiting, but now in a small dark basement anteroom. She is lying casually and comfortably on a trolley, reading something from *Chat* magazine to Marcus. She is probably telling him a joke. She isn't in pain.

(Who is Marcus? Marvellous, quirky Marcus Konig, a leading light at Sturts Farm and their chief farmer. Marcus himself was to die fourteen years later in this same hospital, at only 48 years old, from a rare autoimmune disease.)

Marcus is sitting patiently in a corner on a less comfortable chair, just chumming Daisy until we arrived.

A long wait begins. No one knows it is happening, but fat from Daisy's strong, young bone marrow is leaking, seeping, creeping from the broken bones into her bloodstream. Lying still, Daisy's blood flows smoothly and knowingly on, uninterrupted, round her body. Several accidents and emergencies are coming through into the hospital and it is too busy to operate fully on Daisy, so a stabilizing back slab is put on her leg (a back slab is a cast that can be removed quickly and safely). She is taken to a ward to wait for an operation to mend her two cleanly, completely, snapped leg bones, the tibia and fibula.

She is taken up to Ward B3, a pretty pink-walled and pink-flowered curtained ward almost just exactly like those we had seen twenty-two years ago in St Bartholomew's Hospital, though a little smarter and more modern. Daisy is cosy in bed, surrounded by her colouring books to occupy the time. She is left alone to wait, but as a seasoned hospital patient, is not afraid or alarmed or upset. We are a little anxious, but not at all panicky.

So we drive the long way back home again to Brighton (about a 175-mile round trip) for me to try to catch up on detailed preparations in advance of an important government inspection of the centre I worked in which is due to take place the next week. Later that day Sam, grown up now, drives after work from London to visit his sister Daisy.

Back home I make hasty plans, try to think of everything I need to prepare at work, and then I do some early Christmas shopping. It is to be the only Christmas shopping I do that year. Each Christmas now, I shop early, not to get a bargain, not to be well prepared. Just in case, in case, in case. In case Christmas never happens. Keep calm under pressure.

It never ever leaves you - the fear of what might happen, the desire to leave everything okay because what comes will probably not be okay. Preparing for death draws you from life, but it is impossible to stop.

Here's how it is described in a business book.
Principle 4
Avoid reach-back and after-burn.
Worry, about a future event, is known as reach-back.
Worry about a previous event is known as after-burn.
The two often collide.
After-burn is a situation in which your thoughts about a past event are carried forward and have a negative impact on your current situation. These emotionally

driven processes can be avoided by accepting the possibility of a less than perfect outcome.

Of course, we accept this - a less than perfect outcome - don't we? Didn't we? Do I?

Daisy is settled into Ward B3. Tim always has lots of notebooks - leather bound, with pretty printed designs or smooth ties. Once, in Spain, he delightedly and triumphantly bought a small notebook with the pattern of a beautiful Moorish tile on the cover. He thought there would be a beautiful tile on each of its thick paper pages. There wasn't, and he was so cross he demanded the return of his €2.50. (It wasn't refunded). No notebook Tim begins is ever completed.

In Tim's diary is scribbled.
DB cheerful. TV.

DB stands for Daisybelle, one of Daisy's many nicknames, and the TV had been very expensively hired and installed by her bed. Daisy's nearly always cheerful.

Sam phones after his visit to update us. Daisy was fine but had complained she felt cold when he left. A bit strange, as hospitals are always so hot and stuffy. We are at home in Brighton. We plan to sleep there tonight and set off early tomorrow back to Poole to visit Daisy again.

But, about 10pm, the phone in our long dark hallway rings. It's Poole Hospital. Daisy is "conscious but unresponsive."

"Can you come back as soon as possible?"

"Now? Now?"

"As soon as possible."

There's no explanation. The young nurse's voice sounds cautious and anxious. We do not waste time asking why, sensing there is not going to be any explanation, but we of course we do wonder. Has she fallen out of bed?

I've started trying to explain, Daisy, what happened to you. We have just left you waiting for an operation, but here is the first part of a letter I received from one of your doctors much later.

SUMMARY LETTER FROM DR K POWER,
THE RONALD FISHER DEPARTMENT OF ANAESTHESIA,
POOLE HOSPITAL TRUST
JANUARY 1997

Dear Mrs. Hodlin,

Following your recent letter, I have endeavoured to put together a chronological account of Daisy's intensive care admission from the medical point of view.

Kind regards

Yours sincerely

Dr Ken Power

Consultant in Anaesthesia and Intensive Care.

Trying to make sense of the month in hospital that had just passed, I had written to Dr Power to ask if he could explain what had happened. The wonderful Dr Ken Power and Dr Barry Newman. The Doctor Duo. Always calm, energetic, positive, smart, standing, carefully discussing options, at the foot or at the side of Daisy's bed in the Intensive Care Unit.

Daisy was 25 at the time of her admission in November 1996. She had fallen from her horse and been stamped on, sustaining a closed transverse fracture of the middle shaft of both the tibia and the fibula in the lower leg. She was initially treated with a plaster back slab and a traction pin through the heel with a view to definitive surgery with a fixation device known as a locking nail.

Daisy had a past medical history of a medullablastoma which had been treated with radiotherapy to the brain. She was on Carbamazepine (anti-convulsant). Initially things went fairly well but after 48 hours, on November 23, medical staff were called to see Daisy as she had become somewhat wheezy and breathless and was found to have spiked a temperature of 40°.

How on earth did we get here? How are we once again in a hospital Intensive Care Unit? Daisy is born. Daisy is a two-year-old. Daisy gets ill. Daisy almost dies. Damaged Daisy carries on. We carry on. This is our life. We bring up our children. We deal with it. Daisy deals with it. Until this.

Chapter Four

Independent Years

After school, before moving to the Camphill Community, Daisy spent two years at the Fortune Centre in the New Forest. The Fortune Centre for Riding Therapy, with its motto *'Hold Fast to Reality'*.

If only one knew what reality is.

The Fortune Centre had been recommended to us by one of my friends, a colleague at work. Before this recommendation to the Fortune Centre, our Local Authority forced us through the ritual of visiting each possible placement for Daisy, a dreadful and depressing experience. But at this Centre, individuals are given the opportunity to gain life skills and knowledge needed to live an independent life. Skills are taught to disadvantaged youngsters through living and working with horses. To win a place, students must have 'a love of horses, a passion for all things horsey, and they must be 'horse-motivated.'

Daisy didn't have the former and wasn't the latter. But, to us, the Fortune Centre seemed like a realistic lifeline. Here, she would learn how to live away from home, to be with others in shared learning, and how to look after and ride horses. Competition for a place at the Fortune Centre was fierce and involved another struggle for us to justify an 'out-of-county' placement for Daisy after schooling finished. Then there needed to be an assessment followed by an initial trial week.

Daisy's Trial Week commenced. The assessment report of this week noted, 'Daisy did not enjoy the early start to the day involved with horses, but nevertheless always managed it somehow.'

Somehow Daisy always manages, (even though, as the report continued, 'At times she used her verbal skills to avoid action.') I wonder who she inherited those skills from? Anyone who knew Tim might tell you.

Daisy, fully admitted to the Fortune Centre, is now living away from home for the first time. She is only just sixteen. She gets regular letters from her dad.

FROM RAMHILL FARMHOUSE, OVING, BUCKINGHAMSHIRE.

8th October 1989

From: Duke of Nassau; His Royal Highness TPN HODLIN & WILLIAM[2] The Court Dog extraordinary.

TO: Princess Daisy of the Crazed Elephants[3] and holder of the BROKEN WALKMAN award for 1988/9

GREETINGS O CHUBS!

No horses[4] having crippled you, bit you, shat on you, I hope this week? They have? Good. It will BUILD your CHARACTER and make you a fine HUMAN being.

We have had a busy week.

William can now run in the fields properly as the sheep have gone to be little lamb chops, I trust, and I

---

[2] William was our first dog.

[3] It wasn't the elephants that were crazed. On holiday in Sri Lanka, we made a visit to watch the holy washing of elephants in the river. Volunteers to do it? Only Daisy walks forward and enthusiastically sits on a slippery wet, huge elephant half kneeling in the river and helps to wash him.

[4] This letter was written to Daisy eight years before the accident with the carthorse.

have made another concrete head with chicken wire plus cement.

I have been to London twice and played some cards. I won. I am waiting to make another film and am seeing a TV actress next week. Her name is KB[5] and she acted with French & Saunders in that funny song which copied Bananarama 'Help!' I hope to do some comic films with her like *Buygones*[6], but the other film is about education[7].

Mum said you would have liked to help me with my cement. I will do another head when you come home next time.

Now, little piglet. Write a letter to ME ME ME and William.

We miss you a lot. Who can I shout at when my things go missing? We tidied up the garden. Sue mowed the lawn. It's too much for my sweet little hands. I might get a blister and that would never do. I gave her a sweetie afterwards. I am very generous.

I am moving all the flowers into the greenhouse as it is getting cold. Frost will kill them unless I leave them inside. They look very pretty, and the orchids are coming out.

We went to a funeral at Windsor Castle for a friend[8] who died last week. There were six hundred people.

---

[5] Kathy Burke, an actress.

[6] Tim made a series of films with Victor Lewis-Smith, called *Buygones*

[7] This film was made for Channel 4 with the title *Education for Sale*

[8] This friend (Justin) was the middle son of our very good friends, Hugh and Vanessa. Young and fit, he drowned in an accident off the west coast of Ireland, with three others. Hugh worked in the

We wore dark clothes, and the singing was very good,
though it was sad about the dead person.
I am not dead and therefore am writing to you.
Much love,
TIM (your father) and WILLIAM (your dog)
10th October

Darling Daisy,
still crazy?
dear old dad,
(who's still very bad,)
Sez, hello Belle,
You sound very well,
But sometimes a little sad.

now, young daisy Belle,
Phone when you're sad,
or mad,
Or both, but remember, dear Daise,
We love you and not your moans,
(You can buy Will his bones)
Sam and I miss you, but we're proud!
We've no-one to blame for milk spills,
Shoes around, food spilled, records loud.
But we're very proud of you!
love you
Tim

British Embassy in Tehran. They both know Daisy well and had
seen the minute-by-minute puzzlement of her sickness which first
began after a lunch and a day at their house. In Vanessa's eyes
always I can see her pain, and her understanding of our pain.

Monday 4th November

Darling, dearest, doo-doo Daisy,

So! I will be seeing you on Thursday evening. Hoorah!

Have you got that cassette, *Children's Favourites*? A BBC tape?

It was jolly cold this weekend and I lit the wood fire. William and the communard cats hogged it while we sat coldly around them.

Sam is working nearly every day and is sometimes a grumble-bugger. Sue (your mother if you remember) has gone off to Brighton after chomping porridge. I made her a bowl of yogurt and she made our Christmas cake.

William had a letter from his friend, Fred, at the North Pole. I couldn't read it. It looked like this (paw marks). A special paw language. Anyway, William told me what it said. It seems that Fred got to the iceberg area and it was very, very cold, so he made friends with a dog (a St Bernard) who had some brandy in a barrel round his neck. Fred got very drunk and lost his map. A polar bear chased him, and he found a seal post office to send a letter to William. Now William has a biscuit box 'Help Fred Fund' and we all put biscuits in it. I'm not sure that William will really send them all. Maybe most of them.

All love

TimPaDad

Tuesday 29th October

Darling Daisy

It was very enjoyable seeing your happy little face at the weekend, so I thought I would write and tell you so.

There.

I've told you.

Yesterday Sam went to work, but there was a gas leak at the back of the garage, so the police cleared the area and turned all the cars around. I left Sam there and went shopping at YAWN! YAWN! Tesco's at Bicester. This proved very boring. Tesco's at Bicester has better coffee and buns but nothing interesting except bubble bath which goes PING!

William bought himself a scarf with all his saved-up biscuits which he sold to a Labrador leaving for the North Pole to seek a bone mine.

O miss you. All love

Tim

Monday 7th November

Dearest Snotbag,

What a day!

William and I had our sleep and woke up to a shock! In the morning, I had gone to Winslow for the weekly bone.

It was a large one, with lots of marrow and meat. William was very proud of it. (He made a nice pan of chips to go with it, actually) and we had our nap ready for the FEAST!

William woke first and went to see if the bone was ready, after a little time soaking in hot wine which always helps meat go down, but well, back to the SHOCK!

IT WAS GONE! Meat, chips.... everything. William lay down on his back and groaned. Helpless, I watched him YOWL and HOWL. I rang the police, but they refused to help. So, after I had fed William some restoring cake, (only a little, must watch his weight), we decided to track down the thief or thieves, ourselves.

Imagecrest[9] is now a Dog Detective Agency. Will do anything, sniff anything (or at least William will) and I will report on the investigation next week.

lots of love old bean,

Detective Inspector Tim and Sergeant William.

Daisy still goes riding now in the high Alpujarras in Southern Spain, led by Sarah. It takes a few of us to get her up and on the horse she is going to ride, Peepa. Over Peepa's ears are little dark blue felt cone 'sleeves' to keep away the flies. His forehead is covered with the same cloth with fringes touching his long dark lashes. We drag Daisy's wheelchair across the yard and Daisy totters frighteningly, with help, onto the steps, then three of us help her up and yes! onto the saddle. Peepa is patient. Daisy is closely supported on the left side and the right side. Peepa, Daisy, Sarah and a little band of helpers carefully set off and make it out and up to the track, slowly picking their way along the uneven field. Daisy sits expertly upright, but, slowly, inevitably, on the return walk down the steep path, she begins to keel over to one side. It's heart stopping to watch. Daisy enjoys it, just like she has always enjoyed riding.

---

[9] Imagecrest was Tim's television film production company

Chapter Five

Memories for Daisy

Here are some memories for you, Daisy.

BIRTHDAYS
SEPTEMBER 8, 1973 (2 years old)

A photo. Daisy, in a pale purple smocked dress, is sitting on the back of a man who is crawling along the grass in a race. The man is a friend's dad and my work colleague too. We are in the garden of Tim's mum and dad's house, holding a garden party for Daisy's second birthday. I am sitting behind her. Sam is lying sleeping in my arms, one month old. There are lots of children skipping around. Daisy's fair curls are lit by the sun. Daisy, aged two, is growing. A tumour is growing inside her, too, filling that empty little space in a child's soft, developing, growing head.

After Daisy's operation in 1974, birthday parties become less frequent. It's too complicated and too distressful to create happiness, although we still try.

SEPTEMBER 8, 1989 (18 years old)
Daisy celebrates her 18th birthday with a visit to the Isle of Wight with us and a friend. On the way home, we have a picnic with her birthday cake in the New Forest.

SEPTEMBER 8, 1992 (21 years old)
Daisy sits on a Brighton beach, holding this year's birthday cake up for the camera. On the cake is a picture of Daisy and Max, our dog, in icing. On Daisy's real face is Daisy's real beam.

SEPTEMBER 8, 2011 (40 years old)
Now there is no Tim anymore, but we celebrate Daisy's 40th birthday with Sam and Sue, his wife, and with Daisy's two gorgeous nieces, and our two granddaughters, Ava Isabelle and Amelia Rose. We all (us big girls) have head and body massages and lots of pampering at a local spa.

SEPTEMBER 8, 2014 (43 years old)
A hot, hot, hot day in Spain. A group of friends meet at a local restaurant for a lovely lunch. New friends, many of whom have only known Daisy in her wheelchair. There are jokes, and fun, and Spanish and Moroccan food and sun. An impossible 43 years.

SEPTEMBER 8, 2021 (50 years old)
A catamaran boat trip from Brighton Marina to see the 116 windfarms at sea off the coast in Brighton. Daisy sits on one of the boat's benches and grips the handrail, tightly. She doesn't really lift her heads as we get up close to the huge structures and the intricacies of the magnificent wind farms are explained to us. "Did you enjoy it Daisy?" I asked. "No". I hope the meal before and the sugar free birthday cake made by Ava with the sporadically sparkling John Lewis sparklers and the jolly family company made up for that.

That Daisy is 50 is greeted with shock, admiration, relief and wonder.

Daisy didn't ever have many birthday parties, nor did she ever want a 'big' present (apart from a quad bike). She likes nail polish, a favourite meal like toad-in-the-hole, sweets and crisps to eat, little rings for her fingers, flowers (delivered), ...and joke books.

THE FARM, WEST MOORS, DORSET.
OUT OF THE BLUE. EASTER. 1993
Daisy is 22.

After two years at the Fortune Centre, Daisy moves to live in a Camphill community. This community is a bio dynamic farm in Dorset.

One day, another phone call comes. I still almost hate phone calls, not because of scam calls, but phone calls cut into your life and these phone calls are like wartime telegrams. "Can you collect Daisy early for Easter holidays?"

There is no explanation. Daisy, Tim and a letter arrive home together.

Dear Doctor
re: Daisy Hodlin (8/9/71)

This lass has now been some weeks at our Sturts Farm community, settling well. Out of the blue today she appears to have had two grand mal, tonic/clonic fits, the second apparently lasting at least 2-3 minutes. It is possible these were precipitated by being up at 5am this morning for an Easter celebration[10], on top of probably being tired, and excited about going home, but in view of the history of medulloblastoma one would need to be careful. The parents will be advised meanwhile to limit her TV watching, and especially, to be far enough from the screen.

Yours sincerely
HG
(the Farm's doctor)

Tim picks Daisy up from the farm. It's very strange. She doesn't seem to recognise him properly. At home in Brighton, we lie her on the sofa downstairs in case she gets out of her bed upstairs and falls. She's not fretful, or troubled. As usual, she's happy to be home but is strangely subdued, almost peaceful. She sleeps.

The next morning, she wakes up puzzled, almost surprised but pleased to find herself at home, pleased to find William our dog has been sleeping beside her downstairs too. She is cheery, quite Daisy again, and wants to go shopping. Daisy and Tim go into Brighton together and have a good day out, with many stops for coffee, of course.

In one line, the letter from the doctor at Sturts Farm was to be the basis for many years of drug misery for Daisy. Disturbingly and amazingly, it can still appear in Local Authority documents.

---

[10] The Easter celebrations at the farm used to start with some very early singing to the farm's cows (then all hand-milked). Daisy had quickly decided she would rather be a gardener than a milker.

Here's a note about epilepsy and the aftermath. Again, we took as little notice as possible of this, far too absorbed in other things, and probably still believing, hoping, that Daisy had had enough serious illness: we didn't want any more.

A grand mal seizure - also known as a generalized tonic-clonic seizure - features loss of consciousness and violent muscle contractions. It's the type of seizure most people picture when they think about seizures in general. Grand Mal seizure is caused by abnormal electrical activity throughout the brain.

Many people who have had a grand mal seizure will never have another one… and because a seizure can be an isolated incident, your doctor may decide not to start treatment until you've had more than one.
Mild side effects
fatigue
dizziness
weight gain

(The Mayo Clinic)[vii]

We cannot recollect any further tests ever being carried out, (they weren't) but Daisy is diagnosed with epilepsy and is to spend the next eighteen years swallowing carbamazepine (Tegretol) daily. But she never has a fit again. She never has another seizure. Aged 43, she has spent half her life on this drug. Even so, most medics still seem to resist withdrawing a patient from carbamazepine, which is well known to interact with 1056 other drugs and has a major drug interaction to 165 of the 1056 (i.e. a major interaction is a highly clinically significant risk where this risk outweighs the benefit of the drug. Daisy already takes three other drugs in this high-risk category.) This is never discussed. Other effects of Tegretol may be some impairment in thinking, judgment and motor coordination, and difficulty in concentrating.

NICE (The National Institute for Clinical Care and Excellence) guidelines for epilepsy are that people should be seen by a specialist within two weeks, and anti-epileptic drugs should only be started after a second seizure with detailed discussion of risks and benefits on an annual basis thereafter. None of this happened.

"Concentrate, Daisy!"
This is a refrain constant in Daisy's life. Somehow, she concentrated enough to learn (heart-stopping) to rollerblade along Brighton sea-front, and to ride a bicycle, though our hearts were always in our mouths watching her efforts (or trying not to). Now, post-stroke, being with Daisy is like constantly being on a boat, rocking, swaying, grabbing the sides to steady ourselves and, for Daisy, the fear of falling has become overwhelming. And Daisy, with little fear of anything, has become afraid. It's a great sadness for me.

The pressure, and the interminable risk assessment forms that absolve everybody from anything in any proposed drug withdrawal, takes a toll on us. A young friend undertaking medical research in this area agrees to investigate to assess the risks of withdrawal for us. He ponders. Then he comments that, should Daisy stop taking the drug, he hopes she will feel less slowed down and muddled, and more like herself. However, given how long she's been on this 'chemical cocktail' he adds that he doesn't know 'if she's ever really been allowed to truly feel like herself''. One of Daisy's doctor's thinks it is better 'not to rock the boat' (i.e. do nothing). Carers think this drug keeps Daisy calm and prevents angry outbursts. They are not going to rock the boat either. Daisy is sent for Anger Management workshops. (It was the house manager who really needed these classes). Daisy's not really allowed to be angry, and I can't be, for her sake, or for me.

I bite the bullet; after taking note of the different advice, I am only supported by one lone voice, a district nurse, Maria. Daisy's GP notes about this recording with barely concealed irritation, 'had a LONG conversation with mother'.

When Daisy comes on holiday, I take the opportunity, day by day, week by week to carefully reduce the dosage and to bring her off the drug. All is well. Everyone breathes a secret sigh of relief that they didn't have to do it. Eight years later, there have been no further episodes.

But now, after her stroke in 2013, Daisy must take fifteen pills each day: eleven pills at breakfast, two at lunchtime, two at night. Big pills that need to be chopped into jagged half. Nineteen total choking swallows.

SOME LETTERS TO DAISY and DAISY'S THOUGHTS, ON PAPER

In 1978, Daisy summarizes her family.
Daisy is nice.
Tim is fat (oh dear, maybe, a bit at this time).
Sam is skinny (he was).

Mum is chicken (I am still a little puzzled by this.)
Next it's Sam's turn for Daisy's ire.

DAISY IS NISE SAM IS HORBIL MUMMY IS NISE TIM IS NISE TEDDY (one of our cats) IS NISE TONNY (this cat's name was Townson) IS NISE CHINCS (our chickens) UR NISE WILLME (the dog) IS NISE.

In 1982, a letter came from Dr Sandland (who had been part of the oncology team treating her in 1974, and who had left St Bart's to get married and continue working in Australia).

I am very sorry I have not sent this letter to Sister Kenton more quickly.

Today I started work at my new hospital.

I found it very hard to say goodbye to you all... Thank you for the lovely picture of

your family you drew for me.

Ruth Redpath (Sandland)

In 1990, from Katrina Blackford, BBC Television Centre; 'We filmed a lot of sequences with Daisy, and she was absolutely super.'

Dear Daisy

Thank you so much for being in our film.

You were so patient and good, even though it was very hot and it took a long time.

The film will be on television on 28 October and I know that we could not have made it without your help and co-operation.

Once again, many thanks and I hope you have a wonderful holiday.

Before carthorse Henry trod on her, Daisy had been chosen (there must be something about Daisy...) to take part in a Sunday BBC TV Lifeline Appeal for the riding therapy centre where she was a student. She spent the whole day filming with the well-known, handsome, TV 'Forsyte Saga' star actor, Anthony Andrews who was an experienced horse owner/rider. Most of the time Anthony and Daisy both sat on their horses, amiably chatting, waiting for the filming to get started, and then endlessly and patiently walking up and down the New Forest paths as instructed until the right shots were obtained.

Daisy and animals, most animals, get along. They look her in the eye and they each know something. They are in the moment. She carries supplies of dog chews and cat sticks in the little blue bag tied on the side of her wheelchair. Also in this bag are; a birthday card homemade in the form of a little book made by a friend, Kay (the book is coming apart as it's been in the bag for a couple of years), chewing gum, (English and exotic Spanish flavours), throat sweets, lip salve, a mosquito bite zapper (for holidays), sweeteners, (in case, no WHEN, she has a cup of coffee), a key on a key ring with a glass stone in the shape of a heart, inside which are two tiny stranded seahorses and tiny scraps of paper from Christmas crackers, with jokes.

There's a photo of Daisy, taken in the garden of our house in the country years ago. Daisy is sitting on a swing with a chicken, Cocky-Locky and Henny Penny, tucked under each arm.

Here are more photos.

No-one but Daisy could have dressed our dog William, then our next dog Max in:

a scarf,

an SAS beret,

a knitted bonnet,

a plastic silver tiara,

a cardigan,

a pair of sunglasses.

Max appears in a baseball cap, head bowed, in sandals, one on each paw, red and blue straps firmly fastened. In these photos William and Max have almost identical expressions of resignation and mutiny on their faces (a bit like Daisy really). Pearl, the cat Daisy has now, has the measure of Daisy too, hearing her voice, lying close, but not too close, curious, happy to see if a treat or a piece of breakfast bacon might come her way.

Written on a piece of paper, a long time ago, in her own special style, a question-and-answer session with someone, a teacher? (Read this aloud)

Daisy: i like ET

Who is ET?

Daisy: a spase crech

How big is he?

Daisy: he is meabyom

What else do you like?

Daisy: I like cats

Why do you like cats?

Daisy: picos they puurr

Which colour cat do you like best?

Daisy: totshcils cat

What colour is tortoiseshell?

Daisy: orjin brown blak crem

Do you like dogs?

Daisy: yes i dow

What kind of dogs do you like?

Daisy: I lik plak dogs

Do you like big dogs or little dogs?

Daisy: yes i doo

Yes, you do what? Do you like big dogs best or little dogs best?

Daisy: littl dogs

How many dogs do you know?
What are their names?

Daisy: I now five bogs the nams are willin Josey Bonny toddy holly

Despite the early savage radiation and drug treatment, Daisy is both literate and numerate (just). She loves reading, especially joke books.

Daisy: "What do you call two robbers?"
Daisy will look expectantly at her audience 'victim'.
Pause.
Daisy: "A pair of pants!"
Puzzled silence. Daisy looks a bit puzzled herself.
(The answer is, of course, A pair of knickers.)

Daisy: "Why did the chicken cross the road?"
Don't know.
Daisy: (triumphantly) "Because it got chewing gum stuck to its leg!"
Very puzzled response.
"Do you think that's funny, Daisy?"
Daisy: (straightaway, but enquiring,). "Not really."

I've finally unravelled this joke.
Q: Why did the chewing gum cross the road?
A: Because it was stuck to the chicken's leg.
But it doesn't make much difference to Daisy, who continues to tell it, just her same way.

THE FORTUNE CENTRE
BRANSGORE, THE NEW FOREST.
1987-88

Now a student at the Fortune Centre college, Daisy has 'exeats', visits home, every three weeks. Returning to the centre after a weekend home is always difficult - sad, and stressful. Partings; after kissing Daisy goodbye for the next three weeks we park in a dark lay-by close to the Centre to have a joint little private cry before leaving her, and then take our dark, long drives home. Tim's letters to Daisy flow on and sustain him and her.

RAMHILL FARMHOUSE, OVING,
BUCKINGHAMSHIRE
Monday 11th November 1987
Darling Daisy

Well! What an exciting weekend for you![11] I know you will think that every day can be like that, but unfortunately, it can't be. If it was, it wouldn't be so special. It's like Christmas every day. If you had Christmas every day, it wouldn't be Christmas. "Oh! No!" you would say "Oh! No! not more presents, not more turkey! Not more Xmas pudding!"

I don't know though. Perhaps you would like to be stuffed with Xmas food all the time.

William and I had a long talk last night. He is very worried indeed about his friend Fred. It seems that Fred is a relative, not just a friend. William muttered about cousin's puppies "bad influence" "too much

---

[11] a weekend at home.

brandy" and he told me he must travel to the Pole. Now he is not sure if it is the North or South Pole. I told William he must do what he thinks best so today we are going shopping at 'Next for Dogs - Polar Equipment'. You know - skis, and gloves, food, goggles, food, scarf, bones, bobble-hat. William also told me that when he is away, he is asking another cousin to stay with us. He looks exactly like William, but his name is Ponsonby. "Ponse" for short. Must rush to the polar shop.

All love, Tim.

Darling Daisy
What a week it has been!

You haven't written to me, you bum! I've been to the theatre, been to the beach (to work) and been to the dentist.

My dentist, Chris, made me a super new thing for my teeth. I left it on the table, and William, the dig dog, thought, "Uum, that looks scrummydumcious. I think I'll have a lick... um. I think I'll EAT it!" So, my expensive bridge for my teeth was cracked and chewed, cos William realised it was not scrummydumcious at all, but hard plastic. I had to rush out and buy super-glue to fix the teeth because I was going to the theatre. I was not a happy boy!...
All love, dearest Daize
Tim

The next day Tim travelled to London with a friend. The friend commented later what a good listener Tim was. What? The superglue had done the trick.

Daisy's dad is often away filming. Here are some of the postcards Tim sent from Tehran. Proper postcards with serrated edges and in crude colours arrive in the post. Bright, blue-domed mosques and snow-capped mountains.

Hello! pudding-face. I am thinking of you always. Lots of lovely, lovely rings here, and scarves. Ali sends his love so does Nikoo his wife.

23rd December 1987

Only two days before Christmas!

Just eaten a lot of pistachio nuts and nougat! Yum. Very good, too. You, I bet, are slumping in front of TV. TALKING again.

Questions for you.

Why is the sky blue? Why do birds fly? Why is rain wet? Heh! Heh! Heh!

love love love Tim

Daisy! Hail Daisy! If you come here, you will have to wear a chador like Bibi did. You cover up everything except your face. But women do lots of jobs here, and it's not like other Middle East countries. I've been doing exercises to get rid of my tummy!

lots of love, Tim

Hello my darling.

Another lovely day and I've got lots of boring old work to do. I'll bring you with me next time I come. The ice cream is really good. It's home-made with pistachio nuts. I think about you all the time, love you, Tim

Less poetic or exotic, on a scrap of paper Daisy has written:
FROM DAISY TO TIM (managing her anger…)
Dad is a pig
Dad is a pich
Dad is cow
Dad is a woll
he can fuc of
(no need to explain)

There are some nice memories, but memories can't stop or change this story.

Chapter Six

The Deepening Crisis

POOLE HOSPITAL.
NOVEMBER 22, 1996.
5PM

What has happened? Daisy, who started the day dressed to impress, star of stage and screen, (well, of the local TV programme), the centre of attention, is now lying uncomfortably, untidily, hotly, in the Intensive Care Unit in Poole Hospital. She is now truly the centre of much more sinister attention.

DR. POWER'S SUMMARY LETTER CONTINUES.
DAY 1.
NOVEMBER 22, 1996.
LATE AFTERNOON.

Daisy was found to have a spiked temperature of 40°. It was initially thought this might be due to a chest infection and following some blood cultures she was treated with antibiotic Augmentin and because of her general deterioration the planned early fixation of the fractures was postponed.

Later however that same day there was a further deterioration with a marked increase in her breathlessness and a rapid decline in her consciousness. She was referred to the medical registrar of the day who found her to be cyanosed (blue due to lack of oxygen in the circulation) to be breathing fast at a rate of 40 per minute, to have a fast heart rate of 120 and sufficiently unwell not to be able to communicate normally. On examining the chest, he found loud and noisy breath sounds.

It was felt at the time this was most likely due to a worsening chest infection which had led to hypoxia and that, as a result of this, she may have suffered a fit and been in what is known as a post-ictal state.

At this stage, some blood gases were performed to see how impaired her oxygenation was. This showed a very low arterial p02 of 5.6 Kpa (Kpa is a unit of stress or pressure measurement. Normally this would be 11 or 12 in air). For this reason, she was commenced on 60° oxygen. A chest x-ray was performed which showed bilateral changes consistent with a generalized acute lung injury or ARDS (acute respiratory distress syndrome) which can arise following fractures of long bones due to a process known as fat embolism syndrome. This is where fat arising from the marrow of fractured long bones is released into the circulation where it settles in the lung setting up an inflammatory reaction which we term acute lung injury.

This is what ARDS is. The body, in trying to get rid of an invading object, goes into overdrive. The lungs flood with mucus. The heart goes mad, blood pressure goes berserk, body temperature soars. Now, in the coronavirus pandemic of 2020, we know all about this.

ARDS: ACUTE RESPIRATORY DISTRESS SYNDROME

ARDS, a lung disease that claims more than 300,000 lives in America every year. ARDS has a fatality rate of approximately 50%, despite supportive therapy, including assisted respiration. Secondary bacterial super infection of lung, multiple organ failure, and complications of invasive life support are associated with this high morbidity and mortality. Prompt recognition and treatment are necessary to prevent death.

Despite enormous advances in the development of new antibiotics and in the intensive care unit, the mortality rate attributable to ARDS remains very high, between 40-70%.

In survivors with previous normal pulmonary function, the long-term prognosis is very good.
American Lung Association Fact Sheet[viii]

I am so glad we didn't read this at the time.

Adult Respiratory Distress Syndrome, now known as Acute Respiratory Distress Syndrome, was first described by Ashbaugh et al in The Lancet, in 1967, the year Tim and I married. During the First World War, inhalation of irritant poison gas resulted in the deaths of many soldiers from what was referred to at the time as 'shock lung'. Wilfred Owen describes this in his poem *Dulce et Decorum Est* in 1917.

If you could hear at every jolt, the blood
Come gargling from the froth corrupted lungs

Obscene as cancer, bitter as the cudd.

In the 1960s, ARDS gets another new modern name. The understanding of 'shock lung' developed and it became known as 'Da Nang Lung' after a coastal region of Vietnam where the first major incursion in the Vietnam War by US Marines took place in 1965.

Using their understanding of 'shock lung', the US military were determined to evacuate the wounded as quickly as possible to receive immediate medical attention, but this approach seemed to worsen outcomes and many men died in the days and weeks post evacuation from intractable pulmonary edema and respiratory failure.

A puzzle.

For a time, the military were even convinced the Viet Cong were using a phosgene gas-like agent in the conflict. But this was not the case; the generalized pulmonary edema was arising secondary to injuries distant from the lungs by a mechanism unknown.

In a nutshell: ARDS is the development of a non-cardiogenic pulmonary edema following a recognized insult to the lung[ix] – in Daisy's case this recognised insult was a descending carthorse hoof cracking her fibula and tibia releasing quantities of fat from the marrow bone which leaked into her blood stream and settled as a fat embolism insult in her lung

DR POWER'S SUMMARY LETTER
DAY 1
NOVEMBER 22, 1996
THE EVENING

By 8 o'clock that evening, there is a note that her level of consciousness had improved considerably with oxygen therapy but that her oxygen levels still remained dangerously low. She was therefore referred to us on the intensive care unit and indeed admitted to ICU at 10 o'clock on the evening of 23 November.

On that day Daisy had been
Up for breakfast early.
   In a sunny field at 10am.
      In an ambulance at 2pm.
        In a waiting room at 4pm.
          In a ward at 5pm.
            In Intensive Care at 10pm.

Tim and I are rushing along the coast to get back to the hospital. There is a radio play on about death. Something Russian? Tim says I drove very fast. He meant too fast. On a later, similar rush to be with Daisy we receive a speeding fine. Despite an appeal that our daughter had broken her leg and was in an unexpectedly precarious state at the hospital, the appeal was rejected. Back in 1974, our parked car at St Bartholomew's in London was towed away for over-staying in the space we had left it during the (to us) unexpectedly very long wait for Daisy to emerge from the operating theatre. We retrieved the car from the pound and that time the fine was instantly refunded.

We get to Poole in under an hour and a quarter, rather faster than our usual two-hour journey. We reach the hospital, park the car in the same car park as before, directly opposite, looking up at the huge hospital building, most of its windows in darkness. We leave William, our dog, in the car. William loves the car. He's used to being left in it. It's his home-from-home kennel. He settles down to sleep. We go straight back up to Orthopedic Ward B3. No Daisy. Time slows. We find our way back to Reception and, after some confusion, we are eventually directed up through many dark turning corridors that are to become so, so familiar, to the Intensive Care Unit (ICU).

The ICU is that place visited only by those, all with pale and drawn anxious faces, who know their way here and know the routine to get in. On the noticeboard outside the unit there are cheerful photos showing the faces of each of the staff. They exude some special look: calm, smiling, watchful, full of knowing. 'Visitors please ring and wait for attention' has been added in a scribbled note pinned to the board. A huge NO SMOKING sign is by the door.

Daisy is in a bed directly close to the huge, curved desk of the nurses' station. There are always nurses there, standing reading notes, sitting looking at screens or folders, reading magazines, chatting, not particularly quietly as these patients are beyond being disturbed. There is always a box(es) of biscuits and a box(es) of chocolates on the desk. Above the bed is written 'Daisey Holdin'. Tim never lets them change this... in case...because, as it is wrong, and our 'Daisy Hodlin' will be all right. The devil will not steal her.

To the uninitiated, it's the monitor screens in an IC unit that immediately take your attention. It's where your eyes go as you enter the room, straightaway. There's never much movement or sound from the people in the beds. Walk in, wash your hands, look up at the screen. Now we start to stare at and study the monitor above the bed. Heart rate, oxygen input, much else. But you fix on the oxygen, always. 60, 70% pumped in, 90, 80, 70%, less and less is being re-oxygenated. Daisy is breathing strangely, quite hard, quite noisily. We don't know anything. We don't understand really what might be happening. We are shown pictures of her lungs and our blurred eyes cannot understand the black fuzzy patches on those small lungs. Air is unable to circulate in Daisy. Daisy cannot circulate air. Her lungs are unstoppably stiffening. She has a fat embolism. She is relentlessly developing ARDS.

A helpful leaflet
The Intensive Care Unit
On initial admission to ICU, your relative will undergo assessment and stabilization. During this time various drips and tubes to assist in monitoring and treatment may have to be attached.

There will be a lot of equipment. Please do not be anxious about this equipment, or the alarms on the ventilators and monitors which are set to inform the nurse of any change. The unit can be quite busy at times, and rather noisy.

Poole Hospital Information for Visitors 1st issued 1997. This booklet has been produced to provide you with some practical advice and information when you visit your relative or friend in the Intensive Care Unit at this difficult and anxious time.

DR POWER'S LETTER CONTINUES…

When she arrived on the intensive care unit, she was clearly very unwell, had a temperature of 38 C, a rapid heart rate of 120 per minute with a relatively low blood pressure at 90/50. Despite 60% oxygen her saturations (which are the levels of oxygen in the arterial blood supply) remained low at 85. The diagnosis at this stage was thought to favour the fat emboli syndrome rather more than a chest infection and she was commenced on a form of respiratory support known as CPAP. This, as you will remember, was the tight-fitting mask applied to the face which delivers oxygen at a high concentration whilst maintaining a degree of distending pressure within the lung.

It is very noisy in that room, in an ominous way, and Daisy is indeed 'Very unwell'. How cool that sounds, this description of a life slipping away. (And 'the tight-fitting mask' is not tight fitting at all over that still, small face, and was sliding, half on, half off. Daisy is lying drunkenly to one side of her bed in the corner, the oxygen mask half over her face. Many years later Tim will lie this way too, dying in his bed in a hospital in Spain.)

In an effort to get Daisy to keep her hold on life, we go back to the cold car park. It's the middle of the night now, and slithering on the icy November surface, we lift William out and hold him up by his tummy, while we try to get Daisy to look down at him from the high hospital window. We wave William's paw. The tiny, tiny world of death. All that matters is trying to breathe. All is quiet outside, in cold, grey, drizzly Poole.

… The idea of this (CPAP, continuous positive airway pressure, i.e. respiratory support), is to recruit collapsed lung units and to prevent further collapse of the lung. A cannula was inserted into the radial artery in the wrist to allow the frequent drawing of blood gases to assess the response to therapy. On this treatment she settled reasonably well overnight and it was just possible to sustain barely satisfactory oxygen levels at 92 but this required an inspired oxygen concentration as high as 70.

Abstract (Extract)

Management (of ARDS) concentrates on the maintenance of oxygenation and the correction of underlying causes of acute lung injury. Most patients require endotracheal intubation and assisted ventilation with a volume-controlled mechanical ventilator. Both hypovolemia and overhydration are deleterious. A reliable index of intravascular volume is needed immediately if severe hypoxemia persists, skin perfusion is poor, mentation is impaired, or urinary output decreases. A PAWP (pulmonary artery wedge pressure) of (less than) 15mm Hg suggests a need for increased fluids if CO (carbon monoxide) is reduced; a PAWP (less than) 18 mm Hg with poor CO suggests heart failure and a need for infusions of an inotropic drug. A Swan-Ganz catheter is used to determine PAWP and cardiac output. Management of ARDS is therefore critical and requires an intensive care situation.

Jacqui Beltz and Heather Butler
Second Year Medicine, University of Tasmania[x]

In a daze at the day's events, once more that first night we are led along corridors, out of the big building into cold November air, and into another smaller building. A room with a bed is provided for us. It's very cold in this room. We find out later this is Gala Lodge, the nurses' home. We have nothing at all with us, but later that week our doctor, Becky, our friend from when she was ten years old, arrives, magically, with a suitcase full of treasures. Toiletries, a change of clothes for me and Tim, food, little lovely things that sustain us. We live, no, sleep, sometimes, somehow, in this place, for twenty-seven days. No mobiles then, but pagers, one each, which click and print out messages backwards and forwards via an operator. With Tim and I barely able to function, all our messages are relayed on to friends and family through our very best and oldest friends, Cherry and Michael.

To this day, it is hard to leave the house without thinking... 'If I am summoned suddenly, will someone be able to find my clothes, clean jeans, a tidy house, my will?' Tim and I had made wills very early, as soon as we were each travelling separately with the children. I have never liked answering the phone. Please don't call me early in the morning...or on the bus...please don't tell me bad news ever again. But I know it will happen. The desire for freedom from fear is always strong, and unobtainable. The desire to control panic leads you to control other things, to try to sweep the path of daily life clear, to prepare for the worst. But you know it is quite unrealistic. Most of the time these inexplicable fears are contained, diverted, sometimes talked about. But rarely without your chest tightening, your breath shortening. Conversations with friends are diverted; then composure is possible, sort of.

DR POWER'S SUMMARY LETTER
DAY 2
NOVEMBER 23, 1996

Now into the 24 November, by mid-day, despite maintaining adequate oxygen levels, the extent of the disease within the chest had caused an increase in the work of breathing and Daisy was getting increasingly tired from the sheer effort of breathing with stiff lungs. Evidence for this was, although maintaining adequate oxygen levels, her respiratory rate had risen to 54[12]. When people are tiring from the respiratory point of view, the initial response is to increase the heart rate, at least initially, to try and minimize the work of breathing. It was clear at this stage that conservative measures were not going to be sufficient and that Daisy required intubation (the insertion of a tube in the windpipe) and mechanical ventilation.

Daisy's heart rate rose alarmingly. Sam told us later, it was higher than his had ever been during exertion in a fast long run.

In Tim's diary is simply written: Bad day.

---

[12] Normal adult respiration is between 12 and 16 breaths per minute.

Chapter Seven

Early Days in Tehran

TEHRAN, IRAN
SEPTEMBER 1973.

Daisy is two; Sam is one month old.

In Tehran, Daisy is usually dressed in trousers, bright 1970s jersey Clothkit company flared patterned and printed trousers and corduroy dungarees. There are photos of Daisy in extremely pretty, inherited, beautifully smocked fine cotton dresses, made by Tim's mother and passed onto Daisy from Tim's sister's little girl, but not for long. Daisy will never wear short skirts, miniskirts, all those cute little skirts I wanted to buy her, because she doesn't like seeing her knees. There's really nothing wrong with her knees.

Red trousers, a blue jumper with a red apple stitched on, pinafores with daisies, thick ribbed tights. Daisy's endearingly short, fair, curly hair. In Tehran, Bibi, our helper, ties a pink ribbon around Daisy's head and recites an old Arabic poem, which consoles us that, next time, we will have better luck and have a boy. (We do.)

Daisy travelled to Iran at six weeks' old. Throughout her life, she will journey to Canada, to America, to Indonesia, to Ghana, to India, Sri Lanka, France, to Italy and Greece, and to Spain. By one year old, she has been to Kurdistan, over and up the mountains of

Tehran to the Caspian Sea, and through the desert to Shiraz and the gorgeous and beautiful Isfahan.

Daisy slept through her first flight to Iran. In 1971, there was no provision for travelling babies and she had to be fed in a loo at Heathrow airport prior to the flight and then when squashed in a loo on the plane during the flight. On our arrival, in our accommodation, I scoured *Persian Grammar* by Ann K.S. Lambton, Professor of Persian, to translate, 'These nappies should be rinsed 4 times in cold water until the water runs clear,' but found only 'Commercial relations between Persia and Europe began in Safavid times when many envoys came from Europe to Persia and sought to make trade agreements on behalf of their governments with the Persian government and establish friendly relations.'

With Daisy a few months old, we take a trip in our white Peykan (a Hillman Hunter) to southern Iran. Tim had got our new car by going to the factory where they were manufactured in Tehran and being allocated the next car to roll off the line; it happened to be white. We never seem to be able to choose the colour of our cars - a classy matt black Riley Merlin, a strange dull green Morris Traveller with wood trim (and growing moss), a horrible orange VW Beetle, a tinny yellow Citroen Dyane, a faded matt green Ford Anglia, a cool, dark and shiny British Racing Green Jaguar XJ6, a 'twilight grey' Nissan, a glittering 'Nightshade' Qashqai ('black' says the logbook). Once we ordered a new, smart black VW Jetta, but the one delivered from the docks was silver. "Much pricier, and much more desirable," we were told.

We set off from Tehran in the north for a trip to Shiraz in the south of Iran, our first holiday with Daisy. No Google Maps then, of course, no maps at all (well, there was one of the desert), no Satnav. Daisy is on the back seat, lying on a mattress in her wicker crib lined with prettily patterned fine cotton printed with blue and pink flowers. The drive is long, the miles of desert punctured by the startlingly blue dome of the mosque in Qum. There is thick snow everywhere. Somewhere, we make a mistake, having turned onto a tempting narrow road. Gradually the car gets stuck. There's just us three in our broken new car, in this vast frozen landscape. No rescue service, no mobile phones, not much Farsi (not even Lesson XVIII on Weak Verbs, Assimilated Verbs, Hollow Verbs, Defective Verbs to help us. Exercise 30. Translate 1: I have stood it as long as I can; my patience is now exhausted, or 7: He is so badly injured he will probably die.)

Tim, me and baby Daisy in her striped cream and navy-blue Babygro, wrapped in a hand-knitted, navy-blue shawl, a product of my once a decade urges to knit. I still have, and sometimes wear, a cardigan I knitted with birds and flowers and patterns all over it. Well, they should be all over it but aren't. I chose this complicated pattern on the belief that, as a non-knitter, I may as well peer at every single stitch and attempt something patterned. And it has puffed sleeves, too.

The car is immovable, completely stuck in icy snow. Out of nowhere a troupe of people, men, women, children dazzlingly appear. The women are dressed in gauzy, glittering, fluttering layers of silk and cotton and netting clothing. Headdresses are trimmed with tinkling golden coins. The men and children wear faded, baggy trousers and bulky, padded coarse cotton jackets. A nomadic group. We all pose for a smiling picture. Then, next (from where?) a bus, full, turns up and all the passengers (men) tow, push, heave and wrench our car out of the deep snow. The steering is broken, so we have to spend the night somewhere in a scruffy village room, with no running water, a broken sink and loo, our new baby and it's very, very cold.

It doesn't really matter where you are with a young baby as your world is them.

Daisy plays in the sunshine on a Persian carpet spread out on the flat roof of our house, calling out "agha" (sir) to people walking in the street below. As it is impossible to use a pram in the streets of Tehran, we use our very new (and then quirky) blue striped McLaren pushchair, which is more easily lifted over the jubes, the narrow gutters of clear water running down every street. In Iran, among charming, open people who love children, Daisy thrives, acquires silver bracelets round her foot, wears delicate hand-stitched tribal coats and pretty hand-embroidered hats.

Two years later we bring Sam back out to Tehran too, when he is nearly five weeks old. During that flight Sam sleeps, but now, at just two years old, Daisy never stops tottering up and down the plane aisles, squeezing past trolleys of food and drink. She crouches with us, sitting at the top of the aircraft steps, in the hot air at the landing stop in Israel, (this was during the 6-day war in 1973 when it was not permitted to leave the aircraft on stops).

Finally, with all of us exhausted, Daisy falls fast asleep just as the plane comes in to land at Mehrabad airport.

TEHRAN, IRAN
APRIL 1974

In early spring of 1974, Sam, six months old, develops a small cyst on his neck. We go together, Sam, Daisy and me, almost daily to the doctor to get the cyst dressed. At the same time, Daisy is occasionally being sick - running, playing followed by unexpected and quick projectile vomiting. Vomit is always a surprise and projectile vomiting in a child is even odder as the child themself is just as surprised as you. Otherwise, she has rosy cheeks, is full of beans.

Each time, as we leave the doctor's, I mention that Daisy has been sick again. One day, the whole day, nothing, no sick, but, as we draw up to our iron-gated house, a stream of vomit. Is she allergic to the house, the mountain air, the dust perhaps?

It all seems very straightforward. We are not very worried as Daisy is still, well, just Daisy. She has just started at a play school, the only play school in our area, in Tehran. Later, a friend comments that Daisy did seem to wobble sometimes going up the curved marble staircase in our house. But we had noticed nothing. The American Brain Tumor Association notes that '...children with this tumour may exhibit a clumsy staggered walking pattern.'

Aren't most two-year-olds a little clumsy?

Off we are sent for a variety of checks. Not once is any psychological problem considered (except of course by us.) Eating okay? Yes. Any discomfort? No. Bumped her head? Don't think so. Headaches? How would we know that? Let's just check for a head fracture. We take her, still a little concerned principally about Sam and his cyst, for a head x-ray. Nothing. Largactil (chlorpromazine) is prescribed to check the vomiting. (Largactil was first used to stop hiccups that cannot otherwise be stopped or given to pregnant women to check morning sickness.) Quite an effective drug, in normal circumstances.

At 5pm on 15th April 1974, Daisy swallows the Largactil pill. The vomiting is not checked. Maybe, at that moment, I know that it will not, that it will never, ever, be okay.

THE JAM HOSPITAL, TEHRAN, IRAN
APRIL 1974

Jam Hospital, eleven CCU beds, five ICU beds, six active operation rooms which are prepared to accommodate the honorable patients using modern equipments.
Jam Hospital website

We are sent to the Jam Hospital for a head scan. First, Daisy lies on her back. We turn her gently over on her left side. Then, onto her right. Finally, she lies face down and keeps very still. How good is Daisy at this stuff! The scanner is adjusted again.

The technician comes back into the room and hands us the rolled-up scan. "I'm so sorry" he says.

Why is he so sorry? we think.

We pay twenty-five tomans for the scan (about £2.50) and leave the hospital. We will phone our friend, our neurologist friend, later from home.

Later in Bart's, we are again asked to confirm she had not moved during the scan. The thought, that it might be a mistake, is immediately obliterated by the clear memory of sleepy, co-operative, fearless Daisy lying compliantly, unknowingly, still, on the bed for the scan.

Chapter Eight

23 November 1996

DR POWER'S SUMMARY LETTER continues
POOLE HOSPITAL
DAY 2
NOVEMBER 23, 1996
MECHANICAL VENTILATION.

For this procedure Daisy was put to sleep with a combination of anaesthetic drugs and a tube passed into the trachea without difficulty. Initial suction of secretions via the endotracheal tube yielded some blood-stained fluid and on listening to the chest there were widespread coarse crackles and wheezes apparent throughout both lung fields. She was connected to a ventilator but required 100% oxygen and pressure-controlled ventilation to achieve barely satisfactory oxygen levels of 92%. She was sedated with a combination of drugs namely Midazolam which is a sedative, and Fentanyl, an opiate painkiller. In addition, she was given Vecuronium which is a drug which paralyses the muscles and which is used in patients with the most severe lung injuries to prevent fighting against the ventilator and to enable more effective ventilation at lower pressures.

At first Daisy continues to wear her 'wig'. I will explain more about this this soon. It is a bit skew-whiff, but no one really notices it or comments on or about it. Her temperature was taken frequently and was also rising frequently each time. We looked at the chart - $40°C^{13}$. We turned over the chart, blank, there was no more chart of any higher temperatures.

In Tim's diary: S suggested removing wig. David (one of the ITU nurses) soaked tissues, ice and temp down...Some room for manouevre? Some real hope? Expect vultures to dampen?

We hesitantly suggest Daisy might cool if her wig is taken off. No one had referred to her hair before. It seems such a simple step and almost immediately her temperature reduces minutely. Now she lies with her fine hair damp and darkened. Her eyes are closed. Long, glossy, dark lashes. On each eye, they place a square cut piece of clear jelly (polyethylene film). Over her nose is a rough stretch of beige plaster holding a narrow clear tube in place. There's a bright blue mouthpiece in her mouth, and her face is uncomfortably puffy and turned to one side, a rolled-up towel propped underneath, her cheeks too rosy. A plain white sheet half covering her.

There's no sound anymore of uneven, struggling breathing, only the rigid sound of machines.

ST BARTHOLOMEW'S HOSPITAL.SMITHFIELD SQUARE, LONDON
1975
Daisy is three.
To: Appliances   Office,   Supplies   Dept.   St
       Bartholomew's Hospital.
To Whom it May Concern

---

[13] 104°F or 40°C is considered dangerously high

This lady has had surgery and radiotherapy for a brain tumour and therefore has had loss of hair. She needs a continual supply of wigs about every six months or so and I would be grateful if these could be issued as required.

Peter J Hamlyn
Consultant Neurosurgeon
Please supply Miss Daisy Hodlin with: One fashion wig.

Three is the age you begin to put slides or bows in a girl's hair. Daisy, aged three, is prescribed an NHS fashion wig. These are quite okay, but perhaps hard to describe as fashion. Hot, impossibly regular and even and harshly netted, it takes some skill to plant it on her head, grasp the front, and tug while holding onto the back. The hair is a little too dark, and uniformly thick. Daisy's fair, sad curls lie in that yellowing paper bag marked *Daisy's hair*.

After a while, we decide we will try a real hair wig instead and set off to Wig Artists in Reigate. A day out. There is a great selection. We come out with 'Marilyn, Jamaica Brown'. Daisy looks strangely grown up, ready for a smart day at the office. Sombre, little photos of her in those years reveal a neat bulk of hair and a face that mutinously exudes something different. Real, or human hair, wigs at this time (1980s) could not be washed, so huge bottles of sodium hydrochloride are regularly bought (strange looks from the chemist). The wigs must be ritually dipped in the smelly liquid to clean and then hung ignominiously up (somewhere out of sight) to dry.

Last year Daisy has told me she is going to dye her hair pink. Her 'real' hair is dark but thin. And now, impossibly sadly, with grey and silver streaks. There is no hair at the back of her head at all. Each and every time I see the fragile back of her head, I tell myself, "No hair = no tumour."

Eventually these tiresome routines are abandoned, the solid dark brown wigs and the fairer real Italian hair wigs (Daisy loathes this word) are put aside, and Daisy adopts little embroidered hats and then scarves and bandanas. As no hair grows at the back of her head, we reason and hope, logically or not, that no tumour is growing there either. There is no bone in a triangle at the back of her head. Often her head pulsates with anxiety, as cerebral spinal fluid, not confined, fills the extra space. The thin taut skin reveals the 3-inch-long shiny scar where her head was cut, bone drilled and taken out for that tumour to be removed. Some years later a doctor explored if a titanium plate or mesh could be added to strengthen the back of Daisy's head. It proved undoable, as the fragile skin was too thin, too radiated.

Titanium was first used in cranioplasty in 1965, although as far back as 2000BC a Peruvian skull was found with a frontal defect covered with a 1-mm thick gold plate.

NeurosurgFocus 36
Aatman M Shah BC, Henry Jung MD, Stephen Skirboll MD, Stanford University California.[xi]

Children at school call her "gypsy", and stare, but she sticks with scarves, becoming quite expert at knotting the scarf at the back. Soon, bandana scarves which need no tying are discovered, all colours and patterns; skull and cross bone, camouflage, with CND logos, butterflies, images of Frozen or the repeated face of Che Guevara, first in pink, then red, then green, then yellow. Almost trendy. Headscarves with stars or spots or stripes or swirls, sometimes lined with warm fabric. These, and headbands, go everywhere with Daisy and the number she owns now is of Imelda-Marcos-shoe-collection proportions.

POOLE HOSPITAL,
DAY 2
NOVEMBER 23, 1996.
EARLY AFTERNOON

When Daisy was two and struggling after the operation in London, we had willed her to survive, we had encouraged her to fight, to live, to breathe, to stay conscious. Now, aged twenty-five, Daisy is deliberately being made unconscious and deliberately being paralyzed.

We are taken to sit in the relatives' room, a small side room just adjacent to the ICU. This is a promotion prior to death. Another couple are already sitting is there. They have had bad news. Tea is brought in cups with saucers. Not a good sign. Jane, a nurse, comes in and talks to us. Later, Tim describes how she prepared us for the fact that Daisy might die. I have absolutely no memory of this; I would not, could not understand her words. She had just been explaining things.

A long, long wait follows while they are fighting for Daisy, just the other side of the wall where we are now sitting. Finally, we are allowed back to see her. It feels hopeless but somehow very calm. Now she cannot hear or respond to us. Gone, sedated. We are flooded with an overwhelming sadness, a sense of farewell, but time for a farewell has not been given to us because she is unconscious. Numb.

In Tim's diary is scribbled:
Initially better. Then p.m. D v. bad. 1pm crisis. Heavy drug correction. More stable.

DR POWER'S SUMMARY LETTER continues
POOLE HOSPITAL
DAY 2
NOVEMBER 23, 1996 – THE EVENING

Central venous lines were inserted to guide management of the circulation and a unit of blood was transfused as her haemoglobin by this stage had dropped to 8-3g/dL (Normal haemoglobin 12-16 gms/dL).

A bronchoscopy was performed at this stage by Dr Alison McCormick. This is an inspection of the airways using a scope and she found there was blood-stained fluid over the walls of the airway but no obvious pathology.

Despite all these manoeuvres, Daisy's oxygenation remained very difficult to achieve and there were further concerns due to episodes of low blood pressure. She was commenced on a drug named Dopemine which is known as an inotrope to endeavour to treat the low blood pressure. A further concern at this stage was the fact that her urine output had become negligible.

Daisy's super heart is made to beat more strongly.

At first, in ICU, we are politely asked to leave each time another patient is wheeled in. Eventually, we are quietly ignored while curtains are swished across, or sometimes are not, while messy, blood-spattered, silent struggles take place to try to save a patient. Patients come and go, come and go. Going is death. There's hardly ever an empty bed in ICU.

We sit by the bed, carefully and closely watching each approaching nurse, consultant, people who stand and murmur quietly to each other and try to simply explain things to us. Cautious words; we try not to suck hope from them; we try to stay calm. We read. I try to keep up with work and mark exam papers (not really allowed). Tim leans over and kisses Daisy's little cheek. We continue to take photos. These photos all look flat and still and held in time, just like Daisy. The pressure is so intense you are stunned into ... calmness. I think it's calmness.

DR POWER'S SUMMARY LETTER
DAY 4,
NOVEMBER 25, 1996

On the 25th, I was closely involved myself and I think this was the day that Daisy was first turned prone[14] onto her abdomen to try and improve her oxygen levels. This is a relatively new mode of ventilatory treatment which for various reasons is known to improve the distribution of gas exchange within the lung and Daisy responded well to going into the prone position but when placed back supine she was still requiring 75% oxygen and high inflation pressures.

The prone position

Learn more about prone positioning as an effective treatment for ARDS.

Widely known to improve oxygenation in the majority of patients with ARDS ... it has sporadic use among clinicians depending on the setting, as controversy over its use in clinical practice continues. A recent meta study by Sud et al showed a decrease in mortality rates when this therapy was used among patients with severe hypoxemia (a low level of oxygen in the blood) ... the use of prone positioning showed a 16% decrease in the relative risk of death.... Some

---

[14] The prone position has been used to improve oxygenation in patients with severe hypoxemia and acute respiratory failure since 1974. It has become a lifesaving procedure in the coronavirus pandemic of 2020 for patients in intensive care. (In April 1974, twenty years ago, Daisy had been once before lying prone in hospital in London, as radiation rays targeted her head.)

believe that placing the patient in the prone position is too difficult to achieve.... Depending on the modality used, several staff members may be needed to complete the procedure. Depending on the patient's weight, it can take six to eight staff members to accomplish safely.

Jan Powers PhD, CCRN, CCNS, CNRN, FCCM
2011[xii]

'Too difficult to achieve.' Yes. Each time it takes six nurses to come and turn Daisy who weighs less than 30 kilos and is only 4' 8" tall. The six nurses assemble. Carefully, two position themselves to support her tiny ankles; two more support the broken leg, resisting any twisting, two more support her heavy inert head, threading their arms neatly between the wires clustered all over her body. She is turned every hour.

A pulmonary artery catheter was inserted at this stage. This permits further information to be derived regarding the cause of low blood pressure. For example, it would indicate to us whether the appropriate treatment was more fluid or whether to treat with drugs to stimulate the heart or with drugs to tighten the blood vessels.

Right into Daisy's brave heart, just about beating, encouraged with dopamine.

(A pulmonary artery catheter, known as a Swan-Ganz catheter, was first introduced in 1970). The catheter is named after William Ganz, a Slovenian-born American cardiologist, and Dr Jeremy Swan. Balloon flotation

catheters are a diagnostic, not therapeutic, tool. Its abuse, particularly by relatively inexperienced operators, has resulted in serious complications, including death. 'Swan' soon became a verb. A common expression in the critical care units during clinical rounds was "We swanned the patient".
from Historical Perspectives in Cardiology
A Viewpoint
Kanu Chatterjee, MB, FRCP (Lond.) FRCP (Edin.)[xiii]

How does it work?
A long, thin tube with a balloon tip on the end that helps it to move smoothly through the blood vessels and into the right chamber of the heart is generally inserted into one of three veins: the right internal jugular located in the neck (the shortest and most direct route to the heart, this is Daisy's route), the left subclavian vein located in the collar bone or the femoral vein in the groin. Because your blood takes the catheter where it is needed, imaging is not needed to help guide it, therefore the procedure can be done at your bedside.

We are at Daisy's bedside. We look at her on the bed. Just as when chicken pox invaded her disabled bloodstream and we could not pick her up, cuddle her, hug her during her time in hospital in London, none of her is free of a wire, a tube, an adhesive patch. Through her ankle are Munster like nails and screws for traction. Behind the bed are banks of plugs and wires, thick and thin, yellow, green and black. There are plastic tubes and rubber tubes, plastic rods and steel rods, plastic bags and rubber bags, small trays of plasters and cotton swabs, bottles and dishes and packets of pills, banks of dials and valves, lights and fans, lines attached to monitors and blinking screens. One of these lines is the precious Swan-Ganz, in her neck, floating, floating right down to her heart.

Chapter Nine

London 1974

ST BARTHOLOMEW'S HOSPITAL, SMITHFIELD
SQUARE, LONDON
APRIL 16, 1974

Daisy's tumour removal operation, aged just 2, was
undertaken primarily based on the scan done in Tehran
(a scan that was not available at the time in the UK),
and a cerebral angiogram (performed after admission
to Bart's) that produced pictures of the blood vessels in
her head and neck.

It's not very far, in a small child, from groin to head;
the body is small, and their blood vessels are small too.

This is what happens in an angiogram.

You will be asked to lie on an X-ray table in the room.
The radiologist will put a local anaesthetic in your groin
so you will not feel what is going on.

The radiologist will then put a very small tube
(catheter) into the blood vessels in your groin. This is
passed through other blood vessels in your body until
it reaches your neck. You will not feel it moving inside
you.

Just as, lying in that basement room in Poole Hospital,
twenty-three years later, Daisy could not feel the
marrow bone fat from her broken leg moving furtively,
moving inside her, moving through into her blood
vessels.

The radiologists will then position the tube into different blood vessels in the neck. While this happens, you will receive injections of a special dye (contrast agent) to produce more detail in the pictures.

Daisy's tumour is revealed. A medullablastoma. A brain stem tumour.

The injections may give you a general warm feeling.

I wonder if two-and-a-half-year-old Daisy had a warm feeling?

When you have recovered, the doctor will be able to discuss the results of the angiogram with you.

NHS Choices. Your health, your choices.

The Tehran scan and diagnosis of a medullablastoma is confirmed. There is no choice about this for Daisy. As she grows up, fewer and fewer choices are Daisy's. Everyone chooses everything for her.

We talk this so this casually and naturally today - a CT scan. Who could say what this is? How many of us can explain the C and the T? But we hope that this, a CT, will give, some kind of an answer.

In (only) 1973 Geoffrey Hounsfield introduced X-ray computed tomography (CT). Researchers soon found another type of tomography PET (positron emission tomography). PET scanning uses a radioactive substance called a tracer, to look for disease in the body. At the same time MRI (magnetic resonance imaging) technology emerged.

extracted from Marcus E Raichle. Behind the scenes of functional brain imaging: A historical and physiological perspective [xiv]

Lucky Daisy, born (just) at the right time and struck down (not just) in the right locations.

DR POWER'S SUMMARY LETTER continues

Feeding was commenced. (Fresubin is prescribed)

Sometimes patients in Intensive Care died, and they didn't just die from mangled limbs or spurting blood or struggling to breathe, they died because feeding was not always considered part of critical care. While staff fought to maintain life, their patients were slowly starving to their death.

Fresubin, the drug prescribed to Daisy, is described as a 'tasty liquid consisting of protein (milk and soya), fat, soya, linseed, sunflower and fish oils, carbohydrate, vitamins, minerals and trace elements.'

Nutritional support has now come to be recognized as sine qua non in management of critically ill.

Vincent has emphasized the importance of feeding the ICU patient as "Fast Hug"

Feeding,

Analgesia,

Sedation,

Thromboelic prophylaxis,

Head and elevation,

Ulcer prophylaxis, and

Glucose control.

If the gut works, use it.

Ramathan Ramprasad and Mukul Chandra Kapor, Journal of Anesthesiology Clinical Pharmacology 2012.[xv]

DR POWER'S SUMMARY LETTER continues
DAY 3
NOVEMBER 23, 1996

By that afternoon, Daisy was really very poorly indeed.

Very unwell. Really very poorly. Indeed, she was. And we thought because she had survived yesterday's heart stopping collapse, she was now going, even though eventually, to be okay. So we went to the canteen, we ate breakfast, we paged (what we thought) was better news to our friend to spread the word. We took a book to read by her bed. We were getting to know the nurses. But our reality was not Daisy's reality. Daisy actually embroiled in a huge struggle to survive.

On 90% oxygen there was barely adequate oxygenation and a poor p02 of 8 and low blood pressure still remained a problem. A Swan-Ganz catheter was able to tell us that her cardiac output was unacceptably low, and it was necessary to try and improve the function of the heart as a pump by adding adrenalin therapy. By this stage, her chest x-ray was compatible with a very severe lung injury and this was reflected by high pressures on the right side of the heart. Normally the pressures on the right side of the heart are low.

I see from my notes that the plan on that day was to try and stabilize the circulation with a view to turning her prone later that evening in view of her previous good response. Her go-to situation was sufficiently worrying that I have noted that we might have had to use nebulized Prostacyclin and I have even put query ECMO[15] candidate."

ECMO - Extra Corporeal Membrane Oxygenation. The first successful ECMO treatment was in California in 1971, the year Daisy was born. There are still only five adult ECMO centres in the UK. Twenty five years on mechanical ventilation, CPAP, prone positioning, ECMO, are all things we are more familiar with from the Coronavirus pandemic.

---

[15] ECMO is used when a patient has a critical condition which prevents the lungs or heart from working normally. ECMO allows the lungs to be rested while the body heals the damage.

Fortunately, it did not come to that, but the fact that I have noted it suggests we were quite concerned at that stage.

We live in Poole Hospital. We trudge from ICU to the canteen and back again, to ICU, to the canteen, to ICU, to our cold bed in the Gala nurses' home, experiencing relief to leave ICU which was immediately countered by anxiety to have left Daisy. This feeling remains to this day for me. Unrelenting anxiety. We look forward to the choosing of a meal. We guard the pager anxiously. We get to recognize many doctors and nurses. We stare out of the high window of ICU, the wet drizzly weather, at 'Sunvale', the Guest House opposite. (We never see any guests going in or out.) Over the rooftops, we scan the flat water of Poole Harbour in the distance. Tim puts one earphone in Daisy's ear, and the other in his and plays her music. Is this why now her go-to choice of music is Simply Red and Classic FM?

DR POWER'S SUMMARY LETTER continues
DAY 6
NOVEMBER 26, 1996

My notes on 26th say that there had been a considerable stabilization in the prone position overnight and Daisy was down to 50% oxygen with much better arterial oxygen levels. Poor urine output was still a concern.

DAY 7
NOVEMBER 27, 1996

On 27th the notes report that she had remained stable and was sufficiently well in the supine position not to necessitate prone therapy. Her perfusion and blood pressure were generally better as indeed was her cardiac output and this permitted reduction in the dosage of her adrenalin. Later that day however her oxygen levels were again giving cause for concern and it was decided to ventilate in the prone position overnight.

DAY 7
EVENING

This was the day we got some positive bacteriology back from the laboratory. Specifically, we had grown an organism known as pseudomas from her sputum. This is a not uncommon and virulent pathogen which caused secondary pneumonia in intensive care patients. In conjunction with my bacteriological colleagues, we started her on some very potent broad-spectrum antibiotics targeted at this organism namely Ceftazidime and Gentamicin.

DAY 8
NOVEMBER 28, 1996

By 28th there seemed to be a little improvement and there was an improvement in the chest x-ray appearance, and it seems that the worst episodes of hypoxia always responded to going into the prone position. The lungs remained very stiff to ventilate however and I see I noted on this day that one might consider using steroids to reduce fibrotic stiffening healing process. One would only want to use these once infections had been cleared.

DAYS 8-10
NOVEMBER 28-30, 1996

Over this period, we were very much concerned to not only improve the lung condition but also get Daisy sufficiently stable so as to render it safe to get on with the definitive surgery which was of course the source of the fat embolism problem.

Daisy is admitted to hospital with a broken leg. Visitors, coming to cheer and chum Daisy, are instead directed to the ICU. Puzzled, confused, they hesitate and go home again. Ten days later, the doctors are still working to save her life. Her leg is still very broken.

In Tim's diary:
Op. scheduled. Vast relief.

Henry broke Daisy's leg. From her young strong straight bone, a glob of fat seeped out and into the bloodstream. It reaches a blood vessel and is stuck. Increased fatty acid levels have a toxic effect on the capillary-alveolar membrane, the tissue barrier, in the lung. The stuck globule of fat is an embolism. Embolisms are fatal 10-20% of the time.

Every Daisy turn needs the six nurses, because Daisy's left leg is still, ten days later, in its broken state. Each turn needs tubes and pipes to be carefully disentangled, unplugged, laid out in the order to be re-connected. Her oxygen tube is disconnected. Daisy must be hand bagged to stay alive during each of these moves. These urgent, quick but deliberate moves look frightening. The crude looking stiff thick plastic bag with its wide black rubber pipe is put in place. This is BVM.

BagValveMask
Bag-Valve-Mask ventilation is an essential emergency skill. BVM is a simple step but one that takes considerable practice to master. The bag lies by the head. A nurse stands close and firmly squeezes air into the patient.

In addition, however we planned to perform a tracheostomy; this is making a hole in the front of the windpipe which is significantly more comfortable for the patient when we commence on the weaning process.

Daisy has a funny bump on her throat. She doesn't seem to notice, and we don't either. Others do, often looking puzzled. Later, when Daisy is conscious again, propped in the bed, small and still amongst a jumble of wires and tubes held on to the pillow with brown plaster patches, and receiving food through her throat. Daisy, with a look of intense concentration, wobbles a fork with food to her mouth, her other hand wavers, connects with the tube in her nose, she hooks a finger under the tube, eventually, painstakingly, time after time, she is slowly but surely beginning to dislodge it. Eventually she pulls out and will not let it be re-inserted. Now she can eat properly. In this photo, she has on a flowered headband, a blue rose-patterned nightdress and a cardigan. A broad length of sleek, waterproof adhesive plaster like a kerchief on her neck covers her slit throat, the little forkful of food almost in her mouth. She exudes calmness and joy.

The bump on Daisy's throat, from the tracheostomy, is there until this day. A funny life-saving bump on her neck.

DR POWER'S SUMMARY LETTER continues
DAY 10
DECEMBER 1, 1996

She underwent the surgery on December 1, and I see from my notes that the operative course was pretty stable. Daisy's kidney function had stabilized, and she required no specific treatment for her kidneys in terms of dialysis.

H U R R A H!

Daisy is wheeled the short distance to an operating theatre close by ICU where it had been thought too risky to take her any earlier.

The leg is mended with a long surgical pin or rod keeping the bones in place. Such a shame there is no plaster to scribble on. Two years later the pin is finally removed. The wait for Daisy to emerge from that later, simple operation, which is combined with the removal of an awkward cyst on the base of her spine, is peculiarly more frightening than any of our previous waits in empty corridors.

A few years later still, in 2010, Daisy falls down a flight of narrow shallow stairs and sustains hairline fractures of the second, third and fourth metatarsal bones. These little fractures mend well. No pins needed. No operation, no anesthetic, no drama.

In view of the ongoing stiffness of the lungs, steroids were started to try and improve oxygenation and prevent the lungs healing with extreme stiffness.

Nowadays, Daisy is frailer. Small matters tire her quickly. She is never fully straight upright or gulping in good air.

Sedation was becoming problematic and increased doses of sedative agents were required.

Daisy was fighting to be alive, to surface, to be back with us.

There were obviously concerns for her neurological status and an electro encephalogram (EEG) was carried out (this is a recording of the electrical waves within the brain). This was abnormal...

We remember being shown this flat line, as if there was nothing in Daisy's head. But, of course, there was even then. Despite the print-out and conscious of the cautious worried faces around us, we were not afraid.

... due to changes most likely caused by sedation but did not entirely exclude changes due to the fat embolism syndrome itself or the oxygen lack that it may have caused.

From all the oxygen that has been sucked out of Daisy, she somehow manages to re-oxygenate wherever she is. Tim always said she was permanently high on drugs. Who wouldn't be?

Chapter Ten

Daisyness

Our friend and doctor, Becky, describes Daisy as a quirky, amazing, fascinating human being, but adds that people need to take that ten seconds to listen to her and then longer to re-position assessing her in the context of her personality and very unique strengths and weaknesses, to see her through the prism of Daisyness.

How do others see her?

"Bright, bubbly, friendly, not afraid of anything" (Gill, a friend from Scotland and neighbour in Spain)

"Lovable, special, a puzzle, unique" (Jan, her aunt)

"Quirky, argumentative, cheeky" (L, who has known Daisy for over 20 years)

"Unforgettable, wicked, hilarious" (Jane, a close friend, who first met Daisy on her visits to Spain)

"Irascible little monkey" (Keith, a friend who, much to Daisy's delight, bets on horses)

"Bonkers, forceful, memorable" (Fiona, who met Daisy on holiday once)

"A complete character" (Martin, a psychotherapist). (What a complement!)

After experiencing a family member's major illness, it's a temptation for us who haven't been ill to think nothing quite as bad will ever, can ever, happen again. Subsequent real illnesses and events may be shrugged off, ignored, not believed. Maybe this is why Daisy, pricked by a thorn, will clutch the finger and persuade you to put a bandage on. A cut finger must have lots of plasters. We take little notice of painful wax blocked ears until there are real tears of agony and, eventually, greats lumps of hardened wax pop out into the silver bowl as the ears are syringed. We shrug off injections as only "a little scratch", but for Daisy they never get more tolerable.

Other hiccoughs in life after illness (the brain tumour) just seem a bit trivial.

Slower to progress, in 1978, aged seven, Daisy was referred to a well-known dyslexia clinic in London. The report begins: "Daisy is a very cheerful sociable little girl who co-operated remarkably well considering her somewhat short concentration span...."

That sociable little girl. What has Daisy seen and known? Shiny painted hospital walls; nurses, always fun; Mum and Dad there, but rarely small Sam; friends with bandaged heads. There is a picture of Daisy and Clare, bandages and heads touching as they giggle together on one bed in a hospital ward in St Bartholomew's. Clare is four years old and Daisy is two. Clare, with bright, shiny, clear, red hair, admitted to Barts with a mid-brain tumour, underwent a successful operation. We felt happy and a little jealous that Clare's tumour had gone. No radiotherapy was needed. Like us, Clare's mum and dad, were always there too; John a crane-driver, Linda so kind. But Clare died just six months later, when the tumour returned, re-invigorated and virulent. An impossible shock.

At first, for many years, Daisy is comfortable in hospitals. They are her home. But now, she has changed. Injections, NO. The dentist, NO. Physiotherapy, NO. NO to more pills. NO to more blood tests. NO MORE, please. If she could, she would coat herself in Emla[16] cream and anaesthetise it all away. But she can't.

It becomes harder and harder to cajole, persuade, encourage her to 'healthy choices'. Diagnosed (of course) later, with diabetes type 2, Daisy can rarely indulge herself in anything without a warning voice intervening. Chocolate? NO. Just boring sugar-free stuff. Biscuits? Just those dry and sugar-free. Coca-cola? Definitely not. Lovely thick chocolate drinks with whipped cream on top? Of course not. It's a shame that Sam has no sweet tooth at all, and Daisy has.

The dyslexia report continues:
Full scale IQ 90...this places Daisy in the dull/normal range of intelligence that is by no means ESN. On vocabulary and comprehension (social competence) she also performed well above average and also had an average score on general information. It is also felt that on many of the other tests, Daisy could have performed better ... but if she cannot immediately provide the correct answer she tends to give up.

---

[16] Emla Cream Ad. 'Bestselling Numbing Cream for PAINLESS Tattoos, Piercing, Waxing, Laser & Needle Pain!' (and only available in tiny tubes).

Never give up, Daisy.

...On the picture completion test, that is, saying what was missing from a series of pictures, Daisy gave some very original answers which unfortunately I was not permitted to score, such as the stamp on a letter, when what she should have noticed was the missing heel of a shoe, the key in the lock of the door, when it should have been one of the hinges and a path leading to the house, when it should have been the door that was missing.

Bev Hornsby, M Sc, L.C.S.T
Dyslexia Clinic, Department of Psychological Medicine

It's the path that is always missing, the route to get somewhere or the key to unlock this strange world, and Daisy never gives up that search. She wants to be alive. This report was right, "Prognosis is relatively optimistic".

Remarkably, throughout her life, from birth to now, Daisy has always been supremely, absolutely, clearly Daisy.

Chapter Eleven

Waking Up

DR POWER'S SUMMARY LETTER continues
POOLE HOSPITAL
DAY 20
DECEMBER 10, 1996

By December 10 oxygenation was improving but we still had the problems of stiff lungs as evidenced by the low volume of each breath. We were endeavouring at this stage to reduce sedation and get Daisy awake and hopefully cooperative with the ventilator...

In Tim's diary:
'Response good am. Then tails off. V. tired.'

Vecuronium was used to treat Daisy. It is a muscular blocking agent, that is, it paralyzed her.

... (the indications for use) ...are tempered by clinical concern for... the risk of patient awareness during paralysis. ...A recent case series reported 11 ICU patients who had been aware during pharmacological paralysis. The common themes reported were thoughts of life and death, weird dreams, fear, and resisting being tied down.

Steven B Greenberg, MD Jeffrey Vender, MD, MBA, FCCP, FCCM
The Use of Neuromuscular Blocking Agents in the ICU
Critical Care Medicine 2013. Medscape, Spain.[xvi]

So in Poole Hospital Daisy is both paralyzed and sedated. Imagine this for a moment. You cannot move, but you do not know you cannot move because you are sedated. So which to reduce first? You are rising out of sedation, but how strange, you can't move. Now imagine this. You CAN move, but you are too sedated to be able do so.

There is a photo of Daisy, utterly motionless, buried by tubes, wires. Her head is still but turned slightly towards us. A bare shoulder, a nurse's hand poised over a machine. Daisy has one eye just slightly opened. A second picture: a harsh tube piercing her small throat, a blood pressure cuff on her arm. Wires are strewn on the pillow. Strokable cheeks. A perfectly pure uncomplicated smile on her face that says, I know you are there, I know I am alive.

In Tim's diary:
Daisy off paralysis. S and S[17] down. Daisy waking. Power (Dr Ken Power) impressed at everything looking good. Smiles when introduced David[18] etc.

---

[17] Sam and his wife Sue.
[18] Young and handsome Nurse David

And the next day:
Smiles at joke. Lovely smile. Nods and blinks in answer.

In Tim's diary:
little weep pm.

Now, during the pandemic, we are used to seeing those exhausted, emotional faces of doctors and nurses who are caring for patients in Intensive Care Units. Geoffrey[xvii], a nurse at Poole Hospital, has a little cry as Daisy begins her survival. Kind, clever, committed Geoffrey, always ready to explain what was happening to us, always calm, and funny too. Geoffrey even now, remembers Daisy, and Daisy remembers Geoffrey.

The list of names of those young nurses in ICU are woven into Daisy's story; neat calm Simon, Hilary the physiotherapist, pretty blonde Carenza and 'tank girl' Emma, (why tank-girl?) Jo, Mo, Jackie, Sue, Jane (she with the news of doom) BJ and Gary, 'Dr Death', the young German doctor, who, standing at the side of Daisy's bed one day, in discussion with Consultant Ken Power, moves forward, catches his foot in the heap of wires snaking down the side of the bed and pulls them all out, setting of bleeping, and flat droning noises. Panic. There is a rush to re-connect Daisy to her support. We never found out his real name, but Geoffrey tells me they are still in touch, and that 'Dr Death' remembers Daisy too.

Chapter Twelve

On the Road

When Daisy moves to the farm in Dorset, she begins to travel home on her own on a National Express bus, always choosing to sit at the very front of the coach by the driver. Lucky driver to have such a chatty companion on the 4-hour trip.

When we travel backwards and forwards to our little house in Spain, Daisy always joins us for holidays, travelling without concern on her own, dispatched onto the plane by helpers, emerging at the other end, often alone, having imperiously dismissed the assistance offered. Our hearts are always in our mouths, but we are confident that, even if she finds herself in Grenada instead of Granada, she will, somehow, find her way back. When we do not organize formal assistance, we might furtively whisper to any kind-looking person in the check-in queue to see if they could just keep a discreet eye out and shepherd her safely on board the plane. We never discover why, with no luggage to collect, Daisy is always the (nail bitingly) last person to emerge into the Arrivals area.

Once, Daisy made a National Express trip up north to stay with my sister. A direct, non-stop journey but, in the middle of the morning at work, I get a cheerful phone call, from Daisy (this is not from a mobile phone as there are none yet)

"Where are you, Daisy?"

Already I am working out how I am going to retrieve her. The 'non-stop' bus turns out to have stopped for a cup of tea break. (Of course.)

We think it's time to broaden her skills and independence, so Daisy progresses to a train journey on her own for a weekend at home. I will meet her at Oxford Station. The train will arrive at 6.10pm. Daisy is trained and schooled to get off at 6.10pm. Over and over again.

At 5.30pm, in plenty of time, I am at Oxford Station, ready to meet and greet and breathe a sigh of relief. It's 6 o'clock, 6.15pm, 6.30pm. 7pm. Finally, the train arrives, late. A lot of people get off. But there is no Daisy.

At 6.10pm, as instructed, she HAS got off the train wherever it was it stopped. Where is Mum? Disconsolate and abandoned, she sits on the steps of the footbridge between the platforms of an unknown station and cries. These were days well before mobile phones and it was hard, and very frightening, trying to find out what had happened. Apparently, managing to explain herself, looked after by kind station staff, she is put back on the next train to Oxford from this station, but gets off again at its next stop. Twice more.

Daisy eventually tumbles off a train at Oxford at about 10pm. We are nervous wrecks. She is tired but wants her cup of tea before she goes to bed. On her return journey, she is told to get off at the train's only (fortunately) stop. Laden with stuff acquired during the weekend, our last sight of her is her bundling into her seat as the doors close and everyone in the carriage shuffling up to make room for the many bags, flowers, rucksack, music player, joke books, coats and gear coming their way. Train journeys not such a good idea.

On one of our first journeys back to Spain, (driving) after Tim died, two years before Daisy is to have her stroke. It is a very rough ferry crossing and all passengers are confined to cabins, except for us stalwart dog owners who still have to stagger up steep steps to the dog walking area on Deck 9. Max, our Samoyed, now twelve years old, is plopped into an old blue IKEA bag, with his legs dangling through four cut out holes to be carried up the steps (no Tim to help).

Arriving, exhausted, in rainy Bilbao, I fling our passports into the top dashboard tray (we were in a hurry to reach a green area for Max to stretch his legs after more or less crossing them on the 24-hour sea crossing). We stop in a garage rest area, walk Max, set off, when, on the slip road joining the windy, noisy motorway, there is the ominous clunking of a punctured tyre. Daisy stays in the car while I get out. Another car draws up in a hurry and rushes to help me put up one of two required red warning triangles. The man gesticulates at Daisy, and I, realizing as in Spain she is on the fast side of the lanes, see him half push her hurriedly out of the car and to the side of the slip road. Max, now exhausted too, sleeps on oblivious in the back of the car. Then the man and the other car disappear in the pouring rain, leaving us alone.

We have been cleverly targeted; the tyre slashed (though this was not discovered until much later, when the garage shook their heads sadly and told me the tyre was irreparable.) We have been completely robbed of everything in the car: handbags, Daisy's precious Game Boy, the computer, money, bank cards, but not the roses I was carrying out to plant in the garden in Spain, nor the bulky containers of Roundup to kill the weeds (not permitted to buy in Spain without first attending a safety hazard course.) Ever since, I wish I had listened to Daisy who didn't like the man and who had been strangely reluctant to get out of the car. She also said I should have hit him with the Wilko 'ladies fork' we were carrying out for a friend in Spain.

These days each and every journey is longer, and Daisy is never, ever, on her own. Now, on our trips to Spain, once I understood there was assistance available, we negotiate the airport, often being fast forwarded embarrassingly past the queues and onto the plane first, trying to hurry, Daisy swinging her dead leg sideways and me walking backwards guiding her, holding her 'good' hand, before bumping down into our seats. But on arrival at the other end, we must sit waiting forever until every other single passenger has got up, sorted their bags, heaved things out from the overhead lockers, woken their sleeping children, got up, sat down, got up again, stood in the gangway and finally disembarked before Daisy can make the wobbly walk to the plane's exit door and the safety of her wheelchair (often not where it should be).

I counted once, the ups and downs on the day of travel; get out of bed, go to the loo, get dressed, go to the loo, get into the wheelchair, get out of the wheelchair at the top of the steps from our flat, cling on to railing, go down the steps outside our flat. Good leg, bad leg. Good leg, bad leg (times five). Cling onto the railing at the bottom. (Once, coming out of the front door, poised to tackle the steps, a troupe of Father Christmases jogged up the street and happily zoomed Daisy in the wheelchair down the steps. Only in Brighton. Daisy still looks hopefully for passing help, which is often generously offered.)

Get into the car, get out of the car get into the wheelchair, get out of the wheelchair to enter the plane, tricky walk over ramp joining aircraft to airport, walk (see above). On arrival the other end, repeat, repeat, repeat.

Chapter Thirteen

Sunshine

ST BARTHOLOMEW'S HOSPITAL, SMITHFIELD
SQUARE, LONDON
APRIL 1974

Daisy is two years and eight months old. A toddler.

First, they make a small mask, cast in plaster, of Daisy's face. A sculpture. This is done under general anaesthetic. Next, they make an exact copy in Perspex. This strange and spooky mask now lies yellowing in our loft. I hold it up. How could a head have fitted into this? Looking at the mask today, it seems impossibly tiny. Impossibly absurd.

Daisy puts her head, face down, into the mask, and lies on her tummy on the table. There is a small hole roughly cut out for her nose so that she can breathe. Two more holes for her big eyes. The back of the mask is fitted over and bolted shut. She is lying, alone, face down, completely imprisoned, on a table, in an underground room in the middle of London.

"Now switch on the sunshine, Daisy," a disembodied voice says from the other side of a glass panel.

A burst of Cobalt-60 blasts deep into her small head, deep in a vault under the ground.

This has been achieved by patient, patient nurses talking her through the procedure so that she does not have to undergo daily general anaesthetic.

Under local anaesthetic, the patient is positioned on a table with a rigid frame covering the head.

The Cobalt-60 therapy delivers approximately 200 beams of gamma radiation at the patient's tumour. Treatment takes anywhere from several minutes to a few hours to complete.

Following treatment, the head frame is removed, and the patient may return to normal activity.

As Daisy is two and a half, she is not really able to stay still, alone on a big examination table, in a big empty room, for the short blast of radiation. She can't see what is happening to her. So she has to have a daily, general anaesthetic. This means no food for six hours before treatment, so a very early breakfast. Probably no food after as hospital 'supper' has already come and gone. And side-effects? Nausea, vomiting, dry mouth, sore throat, shivering, sleepiness, mild hoarseness. Even to have four small teeth out a few years later, she has, for safety, to have a general anaesthetic.

These are strange routines for a two-year-old.

On top of the general anesthetic, she must succumb to the radiation itself.

Cobalt-60 therapy is painless. Patients who are treated with Cobalt-60 therapy have fewer side effects than patients who are treated with conventional radiation therapy. On 27 October 1951, the world's first cancer treatment with Cobalt-60 took place at Victoria Hospital in Ontario, Canada. Nicknamed the Cobalt Bomb, it showed that tumours could be treated without hurting the skin. This was the first major advancement in the radiation treatment of cancer patients since

Roentgen's discovery of X-rays in 1895. Cobalt-60 is a beta-emitting radioactive isotope of Cobalt-59.

In order to ease the trauma of this daily general anaesthetic used before the radiation treatment, and to find something better, doctors decide to try a new drug, Ketamine, now known as Special K, instead.

Daisy has returned from the daily cranio-spinal treatment. This is the first day she has only been anaesthetized with a dose of Ketamine. We are waiting for her to return, sitting in our usual place by the cot. She is lowered into it. Soon, she begins to sort of move, staggers up, clutching at a rail, crumples and sinks back down. Now she throws herself around her cot. After a while, some cot bumpers are found and are hurriedly put against each cot side. Now she lurches from side to side, bouncing, sliding off the plastic bumper sides. We try to field her. She seems half awake, half asleep. But at least now she will be able to eat the food she smells cooking. Hospital food can smell delicious if you are not allowed to have it.

Ketamine

A drug with a particularly unpleasant side effect, it can destroy the bladder. Ketamine has quite a history. Discovered in the 1960s, it was used by vets as an anaesthetic for horses, as a horse tranquillizer. Then it was used on soldiers in the Vietnam War where it was known as the 'buddy drug', an anaesthetic that could be administered easily and safely without the need for intubation. Ketamine did not affect breathing or blood pressure. Its first recorded first use in the UK was in 1971, the year Daisy was born.

Next Ketamine was found to be effective on patients who were not helped by normal anti-depressants. Most famously, Ketamine's hallucinatory effects were documented by Dr John Lilley whose experiments with Ketamine inspired the 1980s film 'Altered States'.

Ketamine, Special K, Kit Kat, Special la Coke, Green, Kitty, Baby food.

Special K is the stupidest drug ever invented. It induces a state referred to as 'dissociated anaesthesia' and it is used as a recreational drug. Yes, Ketamine is just like... angel dust, that drug that turns people into completely insane rage monsters.

If I remember correctly...it sort of makes you feel like you wake up in the morning and you can't tell whether you're asleep and dreaming or awake. It's a perpetual state of not feeling like yourself, feeling completely like yourself, knowing what's going on around you, and having no clue how fantasy has invaded your reality, all at the same time.

I remember one night at a gay discotheque in Washington DC.... being slumped up against the DJ booth while he played a Madonna track. It seemed like the song was going on for hours, being played on repeat over and over and over again. In the span of three minutes, I thought I lived an entire evening. I thought I was dancing...I thought I was dancing with Madonna. I was sure I was, flailing my limbs about as the Material Girl kept time with me...but on the outside I was a drooling mess, unable to move, and embarrassing myself. When my friends finally carted me away, I started to hit them, shouting in as loud of a voice as I could muster "Stop it. I don't want to leave. I'm dancing with Madonna! Madonna! Madonna!"

Brian Moylan. online. Drugs 30/01/12[xviii]

Watching Daisy recover from treatment each day is uncomfortable, like watching a powerless distressed little animal. In the end, patiently, nurses have persuaded Daisy to give herself the treatment without needing any anaesethic.

They place her on the bed in the underground room. Then they withdraw to their glass control desk. Through a speaker they say, "Now switch on your sunshine, Daisy."

She doesn't need any general anaesthetic or Ketamine or anything anymore, just the "sunshine".

Sunshine is a strange word to hear now.

AUGUST 1974 - APRIL 1975.
CHEMOTHERAPY TREATMENT BEGINS.

In most cases, chemotherapy is given intravenously into a vein, also referred to as an IV. An IV is a tiny tube inserted through the skin, usually in an arm. The IV is attached to a bag that holds the medicine. The medicine flows from the bag into the veins and into the bloodstream. Once the medicine is in the blood, it travels through the body and attacks cancer cells.

Daisy is so often tired now, almost fading away: exhausted lungs, exhausted Daisy.

Side Effects of Chemotherapy

Fatigue. Fatigue may last for days, weeks or months.

Discomfort and Pain. There may be some initial discomfort when a chemotherapy catheter or IV needle is placed in the vein

Hair Loss. Because chemotherapy often kills the healthy cells responsible for hair growth, it is common to lose hair. The hair becomes thin and then falls out completely. It will grow back.

(Daisy's hair has never really regrown. What hair she has is darker and lovely, but achingly thin. It is likely that her higher doses of radiation caused permanent hair loss.)

Mouth, Gum and Throat. Gum tissues become irritated and bleed. (Any stress and tension now, forty years on, Daisy feels it in her mouth. Dentists look, examine carefully yet find nothing wrong.)

Gastrointestinal problems. Loss of appetite, constipation, diarrhoea, nausea and vomiting can occur. (Hmmm).

Urinary system problems. Severe chemotherapy drugs can irritate or damage the bladder or kidneys. (An already ravished system now struggles, how can Daisy's patient carers understand?)

Central nervous system. Chemotherapy may cause temporary confusion and depression

Decreased blood counts. Low haemoglobin (anaemia). Low platelets (thrombocytopenia)

Increased risk of infection. Chemotherapy can deplete white blood cells. This can increase the risk of infection.

Long-term side effects.

These may involve any organ, including the heart, lung, brain, kidneys, liver, thyroid gland and reproductive organs. Receiving chemotherapy during childhood also puts children at risk of delayed growth and cognitive development.

Remember that while it can be a long road, children treated for cancer often go on to lead long, health and happy lives

Kids Health - The Nemours Foundation

All chemotherapy is most effective at killing cells that are rapidly dividing. Unfortunately, chemotherapy does not know the difference between the cancerous cells and the 'normal' cells. The 'normal' cells will grow back and be healthy but, in the meantime, side effects occur. The 'normal' cells most commonly affected by chemotherapy are the blood cells, the cells in the mouth, stomach and bowels, and the hair follicles, resulting in low blood counts, mouth sores, nausea, diarrhoea, and/or hair loss.

Chemotherapy filling her small veins. A bandaged angelic head. Later at primary school, still bandaged, tinsel decorates the bandage. Daisy is a tottering pale angel, pale as her angel's sheet gown, on a school bench in the second row of angels, tumbling, falling backwards, clutching at the other angels who all begin to tumble too.

Sam and Daisy learn to walk at the same time. We had no thought that she would die, no thought at all. And no fear for her future. Day to day. Day after day. All day. Every day.

On the whole, over the years, Daisy has been very healthy. She carefully examines any tiny scratch and is happy for it to be plastered, or better still, bandaged. A tiny freckle is worried over. Coughs are dosed up. A sneeze mean she's got 'flu. We never expect her to be ill.

ST BARTHOLOMEW'S HOSPITAL, SMITHFIELD SQUARE, LONDON
APRIL 1974

Immediately after her operation and the first collapse Daisy is wheeled away back to a different recovery room, a tube draining fluid from her head, the mask over her face, us holding her hand. Gradually, she regains a steady breathing pattern.

We sit by the bed. Daisy lies still. We read her *Where the Wild Things Are*, over and over and over. Now, I know she heard us. One day, as we leave the ward, as we quietly open the swishing door, we hear a little cracked sob. Daisy is crying because we are leaving. A young Australian doctor keeps us going, always positive, hopeful, funny, and normal, he constantly cheers us up. Dr Malpass, the consultant oncologist, is incomprehensible and frightening, as is the chemotherapy. Dr John Currie, the neurosurgeon, is calm, careful, wonderful.

"Better the knife" he says, his surgeon's pride surfacing. "It was the size..." He cupped his hands in the shape of an orange. "... but I got it all out."

Little Daisy, no hair, pale, pale, pale, but no tumour either.

We did not know then that the younger a child during treatment, the greater the potential learning challenges. Infants and children less than three years of age are particularly vulnerable because the brain is maturing rapidly during this time. How could we ever have been impatient with Daisy since? How does her brain work at all - her mauled and invaded brain?

The Brain Tumor Registry of the United States reports survival rates of 30% - 50% range being seen, but this is only "10-year survival". It is not known how well these survivors do beyond that length of time.

Ten years times five times. At fifty years, Daisy has survived a brain tumour, a severe lung injury, a stroke, oh, and epilepsy (perhaps) and diabetes type 2 too.

Daisy's diabetes type 2 diagnosis in 2009 comes almost casually, and to us, it almost is. But Daisy would appear to be an unlikely candidate, as she lives such a healthy lifestyle, eats the best, kindly reared and kindly slaughtered meat, raised in the farm community. She eats the farm's own grown, glossy, vibrant vegetables, so it seems an unfair blow. So, Daisy, now, in case you are thinking of doing anything to excess - DON'T. No sugary foods, no fruit juice, no dried fruit, then Daisy, you will stay healthy.

Pituitary disfunction after spinal radiation may be a contributing factor, but no one knows or tells us anything, just that she has diabetes type 2. That's it.

But that isn't it. Rollercoaster years will follow.

Chapter Fourteen

The End Nears

DR POWER'S SUMMARY LETTER
POOLE HOSPITAL
DAY 20, DECEMBER 11, 1996

Infection screens at this time of blood cultures, sputum and tips of central venous lines showed no growth. Over this week we were very much into the weaning process and there were encouraging signs of progress.

DAY 23 – 25, DECEMBER 11 – 13, 1996

By December 13, Daisy was sitting up although still attached to the ventilator via her tracheostomy.

A wobbly smile, her legs swung unevenly to the side, Daisy shifts and slithers to the edge of the bed, and slowly positioning herself upright. With one pyjama leg tucked up, she looks round with an uncertain expression, almost as if she wants to walk out of that ward straightaway but finds she is tethered to the bed.

She was now breathing herself in a mode of ventilation we call pressure support whereby each breath taken was triggered by Daisy but was augmented, as it were, by pressure from the ventilator to ensure a breath of appropriate size. Over the next few days, she was able to breathe entirely on her own during the day but only required periods of pressure support overnight to rest her and to prevent excessive fatigue on the respiratory muscles.[xix]

Throughout this period, a close eye was being kept for further super added infections and enteral feeding was maintained. It should be noted that establishing and maintaining enteral feeds throughout was probably quite an important issue in her ultimate good outcome.

Enteral tube feeding refers to the delivery of a nutritionally complete food directly into the stomach. Insertion is achieved by feeding the tube through the nasal cavity and advancing the tube down the back of the throat and the esophagus until it reaches the stomach. The FastHug.

Things continued to improve, and she was well enough to leave the intensive care unit, it would appear from the notes, on 16 December. Daisy then went back to the orthopedic ward and, as you know, continued to make steady progress and required lots of physiotherapy to rehabilitate her leg and herself generally following this prolonged episode of critical illness.

Daisy goes back to Orthopedic Ward B3, into a bed opposite the one she had lain in, getting slowly colder, getting ARDS, one month ago. The ward is quiet. Very few people in the beds can move much, if at all. Unreached supper trays are peremptorily cleared away.

Tim will not leave her, and sleeps by, sometimes on, her bed, to the disapproval of some staff.

TEDDINGTON, UK
1975

In attempt to resume normal life, Daisy, wearing on her head a crepe bandage that now has pictures drawn on it, manages to go to play school a few mornings each week. Here, she makes a life-long friend, Amy.

At this time there were no support cancer organizations, so we muddled on, Daisy as resilient as ever, Tim and Sam less so. Who knows what happened to Sam? We try hard, but he has to be left in the care of friends, often. Just as we could remember Daisy's little sob as we left the ward, now I can see Sam's unhappy crying face at the window of my friend's house while we went to hospital for treatment, or when I left for work. One day every week, every three weeks, we make the long and tiring trip up to London, along that familiar route, so Daisy can have her 'chemo'.

It is now generally recognized that surviving childhood cancer requires follow-up care by an integrated team that includes qualified and invested specialists as well as primary care givers. These teams deliver care with a risk-based approach following a systematic plan for lifelong screening, surveillance and prevention that incorporates risks based on the previous cancer, cancer therapy, genetic pre-disposition, lifestyle behaviour, and comorbid health conditions.

We left hospital with nothing; no follow-up, no systematic care plan, no team, no lifelong surveillance, no back-up, no support, no idea of what was to come.

AUGUST 1974, STILL IN ST BARTHOLOMEW'S, A DOCTOR'S NOTE.

I am sorry to hear Daisy has got chicken pox. We recommend she has a 3-day course of Cytosar subcutaneously 20mgs on each day.

Daisy was in Bart's for five months, day in, day out, every long night, every weekend, long, empty boring weekends. While she was still receiving treatment, it was thought too risky to allow her home at the weekends, until chicken pox struck.

With little resistance in her weakened immune system and her strong red blood cells being blasted and demolished by treatment, when chicken pox struck, her whole body was slowly consumed with spots, lumps, bumps and a rash which relentlessly turns into blisters. It became impossible even to hold her and cuddle her or even to touch her. Her rag doll, frail body loped to one side. Home for a weekend, sent home, we later knew, as hospital was now too dangerous to stay in. Bald head, pale skin, nonetheless there is a photo of her smiling, the same shy lopsided smile, sitting on a garden swing, in a flared blue jersey tunic with a daisy on it and a red jumper underneath, thin legs in dark blue tights dangling, one arm holding the chain of the swing.

AUGUST 11, 1974
DISCHARGE FROM ST BARTHOLOMEW'S
A telegram arrives from Tim, who is back in Tehran, but preparing to leave for good.
Welcome out, darling.

Tim is back and the day comes. We are so happy. On the journey home, Daisy, bandaged, is in the back of the car in her hard, red, cold, unyielding Britax car seat. We are driving back along the Embankment and Daisy starts crying. As we carried her from hospital to car, we had vowed never ever, ever again to get cross with her. Now, to our horror, fraught, tense and worn-out, we shout at her to stop.

Astonishing really that only four months later, on 6th January 1975, Daisy starts at a playgroup.

In reality, we had no home after our enforced and abrupt return to the UK from Iran. Our first flat had been sold. Dr. Anthony Hopkins and Liz, his wife, offered us their flat in Clapham as a temporary home. This is where we stayed for three months before we bought a house in Teddington.

Before we left for Iran, before Daisy was ill, I was a lecturer at Ealing College, now the University of West London, to work on an innovative new project to develop English Language Courses for people who lived and worked in industry and business in the UK. A co-authored book, Industrial English, of this project was published in 1975 by Heinemann Educational Books.

After Daisy's release from hospital, a generous gesture by my first boss enables me to return to work, "to feel a bit normal" again. But you never feel "normal" again. Your child hasn't died but something has. But what is it? The life they might have had? The life you might have had? Now you are marooned in an eternal limbo – a limbo of hope, of despair and of fear.

You do not know then that such binding has taken place you will always be surprised by how easily your heart beats faster and tears must be repressed and how quickly you paint the worst scenarios. You know this is all relative, but that that does not help.

Nowadays there are certain pieces of information that children and their parents and carers should have, even into adulthood, after having cancer including:

a copy of the pathological reports from any biopsies or surgeries

a copy of the operative reports

a list of the final doses of each drug (chemotherapy)

a final summary of the dose and field (radiotherapy)

copies of imaging tests.

The American Cancer Society

All we left hospital with was Daisy,
alive.

Chapter Fifteen

A World That Went to Pieces

1976 - 1988
Daisy from five to seventeen years old

Daisy starts school as normal and at first is lucky enough to be under the care of a hugely sympathetic, intelligently mature young teacher. After hospital, Daisy has a lot to learn and re-learn. In November, she brings home a card with her (two) words to memorise.

(Class 1 will now say the Guy Fawkes poem)
"*Remember, remember.*"
(Daisy)

But when we move to the country two years later, she finds herself at the village school and is, without understanding, described as a maladjusted child who should be removed from the school at once. She is described by one teacher as "the worst one they had ever had". The dyslexia report from Bart's is dismissed as rubbish.

Late Effects
Normal brain cells grow quickly in the first years of life, making them sensitive to radiation.

Some types of chemotherapy, given either into a vein or directly into the spinal column, (Daisy had both) can also cause learning disabilities in children.

This is more likely if higher doses of certain chemo drugs are used, and if the child is younger at the time of treatment. Learning disabilities are more common in children who get both chemo and radiation to the brain.

Learning problems, often called cognitive impairment, may be seen as:

lower IQ scores

problems with memory and attention

poor hand-eye co-ordination

slowed development over time

behavior problems

The American Cancer Society

Children Diagnosed with Cancer: Late Effects of Cancer Treatment.

Probably not maladjusted then.

A consultant psychiatrist at St Bartholomew's clearly sets it out.

.. (Daisy) is extremely anxious about making mistakes and is very obsessional in the sense of trying to get everything right. This is not at all an unexpected response from a little girl whose whole world went to pieces when she became ill...and really has had to begin her development all over again.

After a time, we are lucky enough to be able to move her to a school for children with physical difficulties, many of whom are, of course, very bright. Everyone is wonderful at this school, but for Daisy it brings to the fore the dilemma she is in: not nearly as physically handicapped as most there and not nearly as mentally able as most there. She goes on a canal boat holiday with this school and is awarded a certificate for being 'The best cook and bottle washer of the week.'

Daisy wins a Bronze Bar from the Associated Guild of Speech and Drama. The examiner notes Daisy's performance of *The Little Kettle*:

This was a very carefully studied poem, and you have a very pleasing voice, and very intelligent awareness. Now have still more fun.

'Happiness'. This is a very interesting experience ...and very promising work...and THAT...is THAT!"

Now, half a life on, almost confined to a wheelchair, Daisy surprises many with her abilities. In a wheelchair? We are not expecting much from you.

Tim always claimed Daisy had electrical brain power. And probably she does. Daisy's in the room? Well, the TV will malfunction, china will break into pieces, brakes go off when they should be on, plugs fly out of sockets, electric car windows close abruptly and squash small fingers. Propped up in our study is a visiting card Tim once had printed for Daisy:

DAISYBELLE   MINATURE VISIONARY INC

Daisy Hodlin
Seer-in-Chief
(Mechanical and electrical confusion)

Chapter Sixteen

A Lucky Escape

Daisy is almost a teenager.

Suddenly, another of those phone call from the hospital. Dr. Savage tells us, calmly, that research just published has found a connection between growth hormone and the development of senile dementia and we may hear about this soon. We should not be alarmed. At the time, Daisy was being given growth hormone treatment as, if the spinal cord is radiated, there may be hypothalamic or pituitary dysfunction i.e. disruption to the growth process.

But "not to worry, Daisy is on the biosynthetic Somatonorm, (Somatrem.) We've never heard of it. She is not at risk. We just wanted to let you know," they said, "as you will hear this story soon on the radio news."

Sure enough, the news follows.

Five hundred people given growth hormone as children may unknowingly be at risk from a lethal, slow-acting virus which attacks brain cells. (How ironic). The effects of infection in the 1970s are beginning to show only now (1987) because it takes years to spread in the cells. Britons chiefly at risk are the 500 given the hormone until about 1974. The growth hormone was extracted from the pituitary glands of corpses. Another 2000 plus children had been given growth hormone since the mid-1970s.

At risk, given it before 1974. Is Daisy lucky or unlucky? Now, children recovering from treatment after craniospinal tumour removal and radiation are routinely given growth hormone treatment. This was not the case for Daisy, who started treatment almost ten years after her operation.

The virus causes an illness called Creutzfeldt-Jakob Disease (CJD) which makes victims sleepy and clumsy. Vision and speech deteriorate. As the virus spreads, killing cells in the central nervous system, they become demented and death follows.

Andrew Veitch, Medical Correspondent

Subsequently, one of the doctors in the trials of the biosynthetic growth hormone and who was now treating Daisy believed that it was contaminated equipment used to extract the hormone from the gland that might also be to blame for spreading the infection.

Another lucky escape for Daisy.

ST. BARTHOLOMEW'S. SMITHFIELD SQUARE. 1985
GROWTH HORMONE TREATMENT
Daisy is 13.

This is how it worked. Tim and I go up to the hospital, again. After hours, everyone has gone home, we are taken to an empty dark ward, and we are asked to watch how an injection is given. The injection is given to a toy bear. It is our turn to practise, but there is only just time for Tim to have a go (one) on the scruffy teddy that is lying forlornly on an empty bed. Then, "Go home and give these injections to her twice a day."

We are sent to the basement and wait at the hospital pharmacy. We finally leave there late that night clutching boxes of needles, and a huge white paper packet full of small, sealed bottles of powder, sterile wipes and a sheet of instructions like some special cookery recipe. For some time to come the back of our fridge is full of these boxes.

The leaflet is long. Here it is, all of it.

Growth hormone-releasing hormone (GHRH) with which you are being treated, is found in all people and is important for normal growth. Though the presence of GHRH has been known about for some time, the ability to produce it for treatment has only been possible for the last two years.

You should be giving yourself twice daily subcutaneous injections at 09.00 and 21.00 hours **(Daisy was in bed by 7pm).** The hormone is labeled GRF (1 - 29) NH2 which stands for growth hormone releasing factor and the numbers describe its chemical makeup.

WHAT YOU NEED TO GIVE THE INJECTIONS

1. Vials of GRF (1 - 29) NH2. Each bottle contains one dose of treatment as a white powder.

2. Vials of Sodium Chloride in injection B.P. 0.9% **(this is salt water).** Each vial contains 2mls of clear fluid. **(This is 20 times as much as you need for a single dose of treatment, but this is because they don't make smaller bottles).** You should only use the vial for one treatment and then throw it away. Be careful when opening the vial as the glass may cut you. The best way to open it is to

wrap a clean cloth around the top and then snap the top off.

3. Syringes. They have a small needle attached which has an orange cover. The syringe is marked in units from 10 - 50 units. You will see if you look at the syringe that 50 units is the same as 0.5mls and is at the top of the scale. The syringe may be used more than once. It may be used for up to three days or as long as it remains clean and the needle sharp. Keep the syringe, with the orange cover on, in the fridge.

HOW TO GIVE THE INJECTIONS

1. Remove the metal and rubber top from a GRF vial (bottle), you may need to use a pair of scissors to do this.

2. Snap the top of a Sodium Chloride vial and draw up into the syringe 0.5mls of Sodium Chloride.

3. Inject the 0.5 mls of Sodium Chloride into the open GRF vial. Repeat 2. and 3. once so there is 1ml in the GRF bottle.

4. Gentle rock the GRF vial backwards and forwards about 5 times and then leave for 4 minutes. By this time the powder should be dissolved and the fluid clear. This process should not be done by shaking.

5. Now draw the GRF solution up into the syringe. Expel any air.

6. You should inject into the middle third of the thigh.
   (Only there is no 'you'; it is us who have got to do this).

Use alternate legs and a slightly different site each time. The skin should be clean. Lift the skin and inject as you have been shown (once, on a toy teddy). It should not be painful but after the injection you may notice a little redness around the injection site.

The typed sheet is 'signed' by two doctors and gives their telephone numbers where they can be contacted at any time or by air call bleep. One of the names is underlined, and by the side is scribbled by hand, 'at Christmas'.

WHAT? HELP!

This morning and nightly ritual filled my mind with foreboding each day at work. Open the vial, fill the syringe, make up the mixture; choose the spot in your child's soft skin to inject. Stab or plunge? Do it slowly or quickly? Concentrate yourself or concentrate on your child? Do it day after day, twice a day.

One of our good friends bravely invites Daisy to stay for a weekend. I've never asked how she felt as we sent Daisy on her way, complete with pyjamas, CD player, discs, colouring pens and pencils, vials and powder and syringes, and my casual instructions to Chris how to make up the solution and give the injections. Nonetheless, she did it all.

Soon Daisy becomes impatient with everyone's nervousness, takes the needle, sticks it into the same spot, same leg each time (between three freckles on her thigh) and does it herself. Next, any and every visitor to our house is invited to come upstairs and watch her do it. She takes great pleasure in innocently inviting any of our friends unlucky enough to be visiting us the time, if "you'd like to see me doing my injection".

But, in reality, this is all too late for Daisy, because treatment to the base of her spine will have already fused the bones.

Daisy is 4' 8'', pretty, blue eyes, in proportion. Lucky girl.

LIFE AFTER DISCHARGE
1975 -1978

Chemotherapy treatment soon begins to regularize. Every third week we made a trip up to London. Our routine becomes: play school, walks in the park, tea with friends, abandon Sam for the day, drive to London, spend six hours at hospital.

In the 1960s, medical oncology did not exist as a clinical specialty. A major breakthrough was the discovery of the activity of plant alkaloids from vinca roses. Dr Howard Skipper, a mathematical biologist, put forward what was called the "Cell Kill" hypothesis. This was that a given dose of a drug killed a constant fraction of tumour cells, not a constant number. Therefore, success would depend on the total number of tumour cells present at the beginning of each treatment. Research with children with leukemia with a programme known as VAMP (Vincristine, Amethopterin, 6-Mercaptopurine, and Prednisolone) showed an increase in the remission rate.[xx]

That is what Daisy had, Vincristine. It sounds as it is; sharp, glittering, potent, dangerous. It does the job. It affects all fast-growing cells, cancer cells and normal cells. (There are quite a few fast-growing cells in fast growing nearly three-year-olds.) The medicine is given into a vein. The medication will make your hair fall out (if it hasn't already done so.)

One day at junior school there is going to be a sponsored walk. Daisy gets lots and lots of sponsors to support her, and mostly payment up front, for her anticipated slow walk, once, maybe twice, round the school playing field. Except from the judge who lives in our village, who firmly and correctly refuses to pay anything until the walk is completed, although of course he does sponsor her. On a late Saturday afternoon, the school field has emptied, but Daisy is still there, trundling round and round the field long after most have gone home. She completes twenty-six laps. We do not dare go back to the judge, or to anyone else who generously pledged £2 for the anticipated completion of one, or with luck two, laps.

One day, the district nurse comes on a routine house call on Daisy and Sam. As she walks away down the path, she turns. "Of course, you know Sam has some irregularity in his heart?"

We are stunned. No, we didn't know. Daisy was alive, almost dead, alive...she could do anything and still be okay. Cross the road, climb a wall, sit on a wall, sit by an open upstairs window - it had to be impossible that anything could happen to Sam. But now it was. Sometimes, a heart murmur is heard in young children. Perhaps after exercise, the heart is beating fast and the blood flow gets faster and noisier. After another test, no further problem is found. Now I know Sam has a very strong heart that needs to beat for us all.

Then Sam has to have an operation to correct a lazy eye. We aren't at all worried (I think we should have been) and he only seems to remember the excitement of his taxi ride to hospital and back home (in pyjamas and dressing gown to Bart's again) with Tim.

Sam is soon in another hospital. This time he has on a huge white gown, tied at the back, and a too big paper hat. He is standing with his back against the double exit doors of a small operating room. Facing him is Daisy, lying on her side on a high operating bed, me holding her bald head, while a cut at the back is stitched. Sam is sweating and slowly squeezes himself backwards and slides out of the door into the corridor. He is only five, so we all had had to go to hospital together as Tim was abroad working.

Daisy and Sam are playing. Sam is at the top of the stairs at home in Teddington, and Daisy is sitting at the bottom. Sam drops the scissors he's got in his hand and they fall down, bounce and glance off Daisy's head. She's crying a bit. I pick her up and have a moment of puzzlement that there is no blood, but her head is wet. It's clear cerebral spinal fluid spurting from where she has no bone at the back of her head. Head wrapped in a grabbed tea towel, we drive to hospital, where the cut is soon stitched. Stitches threaded delicately on her paper-thin scalp skin.

Daisy doesn't remember any of this although she does clearly seem to remember (and has the scar to prove it) that, when chased by Sam through our kitchen, she slipped and fell into the cat's orange-box bed basket by the Aga, cutting her head on a rough edge (not at the back this time, and not badly.)

1994. Tim is away again, filming in Tehran, Iran.

Friday, 10th June 1994.
Darling Daisy,
It's very, very hot here.

I have a room full of flowers and a machine which cools the air.

My new hotel is full of mirrors which are painted and is nice and small.

There are three little restaurants near me, and I have a big fat melon in the fridge.

I went to see my dog in Tehran called Soltan (remember I looked after him two years ago). He yipped and cried when he saw me and played. He bites everyone else!

IO, miss you!!
All love
your Papa, Tim

Chapter Seventeen

Traveller's Tales

1996 & 1999 FRANCE and SPAIN
1997 INDONESIA
2000 CANADA
2001 GHANA
2002 INDIA
2003 SRI LANKA
2004 GREECE & AUSTRALIA
2005 ITALY
2007 and every year since, ANDALUCIA, SPAIN.

Visiting our friends Hugh and Vanessa in France, Daisy takes charge of the lawnmower and cuts the grass at their house. Tim takes her for a trip in a small dinghy, 'The Nasty Upset', down the river near the house. (Round and round really, more than down.)

At a Eurocamp in Spain, she rides round and round the campsite on a bike, buys a small surfboard, swims in the pool and in the river and floats in the sea (prone again), scuba mask and snorkel on, gazing beneath the water. She sweeps and cleans and washes up for the tent - the best bottle and washer-up.

Less than a year after our time in the ICU in Poole Hospital, we spend Christmas visiting our friend who works in Indonesia. In Aquarius Megastore in downtown Djakarta, Daisy buys *Spiceworld*, Bonnie Tyler, Puff Daddy & Family, Ian Drury, Eric Clapton and Beethoven cassettes and the first NOW tapes. We buy a huge, dark brown, glazed bamboo birdcage.

There is only room for Daisy and me and the birdcage in the bicycle *samlor*. Tim is left to follow behind in a more conventional taxi.

That evening, the Pretty Ida and Ruby the Fat Domino are the entertainers at the restaurant, Night of a Hundred Spices. Daisy homes in to take a photo of a bunch of kittens hiding under baskets in the market. Each scrapbook of holiday photos has cats in baskets or boxes, or plant pots and troupes of abandoned dogs on street corners or in compounds. Up country in Lombok, she is called forward to be blessed in a special Hindu ceremony. She sits in her red shorts and T-shirt, a lace cloth tied around her waist and a silky ribbon round her head. Her leg, with the long fixing pin still inside from knee to ankle, is stuck out to the side. Her arms are covered in silver bracelets and plaited strands of coloured wool. She holds out her hands, palms upwards, and is blessed.

Time, the years, are ticking by.

Fit and happy, on holiday with us in Australia, Daisy and I join a climb over Sydney Harbour Bridge. We, the climbers, are all clad in khaki boiler suits and bright blue baseball hats with "I climbed Sydney Bridge"(optimistic) stitched on the front. Tim opts out of this adventure with the excuse that he will film us, from safety below. As the smallest, shortest person in the group, Daisy is designated leader and proceeds to walk smartly straight up, along and over the bridge, whacking her lanyard through the railings with ease. The group try to keep up without too much looking down.

Then we drive 1700 miles to Ulladulla, to the Snowy Mountains, to Wagga Wagga, Katoomba, Huskisson, watching out for alligator weed in the canal at the Horseshoe Motor Village trailer park and driving through clouds of locusts which spatter the windscreen on the road back to Sydney. Daisy buys a hat with corks to keep away the unstoppable, persistent flies. We discover our first compost loo. Our saved up one pennies are always spent on Christmas Day cocktails. This year, we drink our cocktails at a swimming pool bar. We swim in the sea pool at Bondi Beach, eat our sea food picnic on the grass and see *Meet the Fockers* at the cinema in Bondi Junction before coming home on the bus. Christmases are improving.

In Sri Lanka, we feel lucky to be offered the nicest two rooms at the *Hibiscus Beach,* Kalutara. Daisy's, at the end, is right next to the beach and ours is next door. One year later, that hotel and our rooms will be completely destroyed in the 2004 Boxing Day tsunami.

On Christmas Day, Daisy dances round the pillars in the open-air dining room of the hotel with Paul, a fellow traveller, and drinks a Christmas pina colada. The menu that night is,

A cocktaile
sanswhiches°
boilled lobster
curds and trickle, followed by plump pudding

We set off to Pathi's Dance Show. The show ends with number 10 in the programme:

'A group dance; 10 males, village damset(l)s, dri(u)mmers, all in unique harmony' and number 11

'Fire Walking,' - in brackets, '(Outside)'. We all sit dutifully round at a safe distance and watch. Daisy, camera in hand steps right in and among the tranced fire dancers and the fire and takes some wonderful close-up photos.

On a day trip to Galle, we take a trip in a glass-bottomed boat. This sounds romantic. The boat is a wooden rowing boat. The glass bottom is a piece of rough, thick glass stuck into an uneven square under our (wet) feet. Tim films two huge water monitors and a baby crocodile with its little eyes just bulging up to the surface. The hotel provides the usual package lunch - white cheese triangular sandwiches, two sweet, sweet bananas, two hard-boiled eggs, all in a collapsing cardboard box. Daisy soon develops a very expensive stomach-ache, as the only loo is in a gem shop where we buy a silver shiny, sapphire ring, a silver gold rimmed sapphire ring, and for Daisy, moonstone earrings (plus two ginger beers...for the stomachache).

In every scrapbook of every holiday, there she is, the complete traveller; boots, trousers, long, long shorts or wide culottes, bright tee shirts with crazy logos and writing, floppy hat over coloured scarves, bangles, sunglasses, camera slung over one shoulder. A good tourist, Daisy loves museums in particular. Visiting one (religious) museum in Italy, Tim and I give up after an hour or so and go for a coffee nearby. Daisy emerges from the museum almost an hour later - she has carefully considered each and every painting (mostly of Jesus, crucified).

There's a photo of a cafe on a street corner in Ceret, France. Daisy is sitting in the chair on the corner, and she has never forgotten the lorry that, in turning the corner " tried to run me over". Underneath a leaflet stuck in the scrapbook of the Carcassonne museum of *Inquisition et Instruments de Torture,* Tim has wryly written in gold pen, *Carcassonne seems just right for Daisy* ...

In every scrapbook, there are her drawings too. Sitting by the hotel pool, headphones on, singing, pen in hand, drawing and colouring. Daisy has drawn; two (empty) sun beds, two stick figures, one male, one female, floating, hands held, in the pool, two neat rows of palm trees, a wooden fence. She has carefully copied the notice board:

we reserve the right to ban from

diving or bombing strictly no boogie boards

Daisy has signed her drawing, 'DH'.

In India, we discover the hotel we have chosen will be the furthest one the bus from the airport will reach. We are finally decanted, and our little group is left a little bemused on the roadside. No sight of any hotel. A boatman appears. We are waved off the road and down a steep flight of uneven concrete steps to the riverbed. A small boat, on which there are three white plastic unsecured garden chairs, pulls up. We are sped down the river to our destination, Poovar. We save a paper napkin from our place, Wilson Beach Resort, Poovar, Thiruvananthapuram, one of the thousands of napkins collected all over the world.

Wilson Beach Resort no longer exists; it was sold on soon after we stayed there, perhaps because, as we sat in the cool one evening by the pool, we watched Mr. Wilson, the owner, running down the creaking wooden jetty, pursued by Mrs. Wilson, shouting angrily, clutching a knife.

A trip to see the mangrove swamps ended up with our apprentice boatman and us stuck for over half an hour – in a mesh of narrow mangrove channels and sand – despite our being assured 'Boatmen are thoroughly familiar with the route'.

In Tamale, northern Ghana, Daisy and I have our hair plaited in a hot little room at the back of a hot little house (the hairdresser's). Daisy looks pretty; I look hideous. We take a trip to see the slave castles, St George's Castle at Elmina (previously the Gold Coast). Daisy is very solemn, impressed, shocked. She stands, in a red tee shirt and flared culottes. With arms outstretched, she is only just able to touch the cool, dark, white stone walls of the arched castle window, high over the sea, the 'Door of No Return' through which slaves were dispatched to their fate by the Dutch.

In beautiful vivid Bali, we hire a car and travel up country, through small bright green curved rice paddy fields fringed with palm trees, staying in a deserted old palace and swimming, just us, in the green water in the ornamental royal pool.

In Djakarta, Tim buys us both a Christmas present. A massage. The massage is outside, on beds on a roof top terrace, followed by a soak in a bath completely filled with flower petals. However, none of us much like the fierce monkeys in the Monkey Forest in Ubud, bounding over to us, their eyes on Daisy's banana, and clinging on and scratching us.

Chapter Eighteen

The World is Changing

ÓRGIVA, ANDALUCIA, SPAIN
DECEMBER 31, 2009

Daisy spends the Christmas holidays with us at our other home in Spain. We all pick our olives. Daisy uses a little red plastic fork, a child size rake, to scrape the ripe, black olives from each branch. She comes to the mill and peers in the huge shiny containers churning and crushing the olives into a pink pulp, and then into thick yellow oil.

Soon, it's time to take her back to her 'home' on the farm in Dorset, and to attend her annual review meeting. Tim is going with her this time, but he is not very well. A bit distant. Their flight is late at night, so we spend the evening before going to the airport passing time just watching TV. Tim and Daisy lie on the sofa, on their stomachs, both propped up on one elbow. We set off for the airport close to midnight. Tim is too ill, (we did not know how ill he was) but is concentrated on making the journey. I hardly dare look at them both as they disappear through the airport check-in. I drive back to our house, and next day, walk Max, clean the house, phone home. Daisy answers. At first it seems normal that Daisy says Tim is asleep, so Daisy and I chat on the phone. On the third phone call, Daisy tells me Tim is still sleeping.

"Put the phone to his ear," I say.

There is no sound except a low mumble.

Once again, with great good fortune, I am able to get hold of our childhood doctor friend. The next phone call is from her. She is in our flat, suppressing panic, supervising the paramedics who are trying to squeeze a stretcher round the corner of the small back room study which doubles as Daisy's bedroom. Daisy goes in the ambulance with Tim to hospital, and stays there with him, sitting by his bed all night until Sam, rushing from London, reaches the hospital in the early morning.

Daisy has always been there in everyone else's crisis, but when Tim dies a year later, in hospital, in Spain she is very clear, that NO, she does not now want to go and see him again after our visit the previous night, not alive, one last time. She says, for some while after, and still now, "But he said, "See you in the morning,"" and he never did."

NERJA CAVES, ANDALUCIA, SOUTHERN SPAIN.
2012

Daisy and I, now without Tim, spend our holiday days like this - sleeping in the garden yurt, mosquito nets fluttering. It's very quiet and shady and cool in the early mornings. We walk up the path from one terrace to the next, to the cool patio close to the house for breakfast.

Daisy enjoys sitting outside, under blue skies in the shade of the olive trees, opposite the gate, watching the world go by. It's not a very busy world there; a neighbour calls "Hola!" over the gate. The 'gaucho' clanks by on his rotavator. The goats come and go. We chase away the ones climbing up and bending the bamboo fence as they try to nibble our leaves and flowers.

One hot day, we drive to the coast to call in on friends, and, for the first time, to visit the famous Nerja caves. It's so hot there that Daisy shelters in the cool while I queue for entrance tickets.

The Caves of Nerja are a series of caverns close to the town of Nerja, near Malaga.

These huge caverns stretch for almost 5 kilometres. Inside is the world's largest stalactite, a 32-metre frozen column. Concerts are regularly held in one of the chambers, which form a natural amphitheatre.

The story is that the caves were discovered by children hunting for bats in a pothole known locally as 'la Mina'. The children dislodged stalactites at the entrance to get inside and, once in, went down into a huge cavern where they discovered skeletons and ceramic pottery.

The caves are big, and deliciously cool. Steep stone steps lead from one area to the next. Daisy is very slow, stopping all the time and gazing around. Just like Tim, I thought. Tim, suffering badly from COPD (Chronic Obstructive Pulmonary Disease), was always stopping to try and catch a breath, and to gaze around.

Daisy does seem very tired, but it is very hot, often 40°C and more. (I learn later that because of a misunderstanding, Daisy had missed a vital blood test scheduled prior to this holiday. This blood test might have picked up her scary anaemia and accompanying tiredness. And was it I still wonder, a warning of what was coming?)

The holiday ends. Daisy is put on the plane, on her own now, and arrives safely back in Bournemouth. It has been our first holiday together in Spain after Tim died there, two years before. Soon I return home too and arrange to visit Daisy the next weekend.

I'm on a busy noisy Brighton bus. A missed call. Two missed calls. The next time, I can just hear the phone call. It's Georgina.

"It's good news and bad news," says Georgina.

My heart leaps. What was the good news?

Georgina and Tim W live next door to Daisy, next door being an adjoining door in the hall, and know her well. They have been off duty, but have come home to hear that, getting up after a post lunch snooze, Daisy got out of bed and then sank inexplicably to the floor.

Within moments she is okay. Georgina, however, trained as a nurse, is cautious, worried. They drive straight to the nearest hospital in Bournemouth. In the car, Daisy is as chatty as ever.

This time, I know. I pack a few things and take Max with me in the car down along the coast again, straight to the hospital. Not Poole Hospital, but to Bournemouth, which is nearer. This time, seventeen years after that other drive, there is no Tim with me and the silence is frightening. I have to find the hospital, as I have never been there before.

Chapter Nineteen

A World Falls Apart

ROYAL BOURNEMOUTH & CHRISTCHURCH HOSPITAL.
SEPTEMBER 22, 2012
Daisy is 41.

Daisy is in the Stroke Unit, in a corner bed. She's moving and talking. It's a Saturday afternoon. The notes read, 'usually able to walk unaided, now very wobbly, unable to walk. Admit.'

Daisy's next stretch of life is looking very wobbly indeed. She has had an acute MCA territory infarct.

Middle Cerebral Artery strokes damage the parietal and temporal lobes in the non-language right hemisphere and produce severe defect in visuospatial conceptualization. These patients neglect the left side of their own body and of their world. They may deny their left limbs are paralyzed or even deny their left arm or leg belongs to them. They may have major problems in putting on clothes, an activity that requires understanding 3-D visuospatial relationships. They often appear emotionally blunted, dull, inattentive, apathetic or confused.
American Stroke Association

In 1996, in Poole Hospital, we started to take photos (on a camera) of Daisy. We had no idea why we started to do this, perhaps it was the sense that this would be our last and final chance to capture her. Two books of these photographs are the poignant record of her struggle to live. These books connect Daisy to that time too. In Bournemouth hospital, one day after admission, Daisy is again helpless in a bed. A flurry of people surrounds her as, in shiny slippery pink pajamas, she is awkwardly lifted, swaying up above the bed on an ugly sling hoist.

'Mother took photograph when pt. was lifted, frown the notes. The next page, in much darker, firmer handwriting reads, Written in retrospect. Informed that taking photos is not allowed in the ward or hospital. They should have asked permission from both staff and patient (this patient is our daughter, Daisy) before taking photos and also if they really needed to, the therapist can do this for them. Informed (me) we don't allow photos taken to protect patient's privacy and dignity and that's the highest priority in caring for patients.'

Here, in their misguided notes, is the essence of the care in the stroke unit that is to follow in the disjointed days after the fateful Saturday, that the highest priority is to justify every action in case...in case...in case and is not to care for patients. Therapists are many but always busy somewhere else. Nurses, when they can be stopped, refer you to another nurse. The voices on the ward calling 'Nurse, Nurse, Nurse,' of those trapped figures in bed fruitlessly pressing the call buzzer so they can preserve their dignity, do not seem to count. Struck bluntly from their lives, patients, evading death, begin their long wait for life to resume, somehow.

Daisy's notes are filled with what has not been achieved, 'not formally assessed as drowsy', or they re-iterate the past history, over and over again, each version, like Chinese whispers, a little different. In page after page is scrawled, (in case…) 'history from mother'.

Assessing a stroke patient's comprehension goes like this:

River Scene

Show patient card with river scene.

Say, "Look at the picture. Listen carefully to what is said and point to the things I tell you to."

Score 1 for each correctly performed. If instructions require repeating, score as error.

Instructions

Point to a boat

Point to the tallest tree

Point to the man and point to the dog.

Point to the man's left leg and then to the canoe.

Before pointing to a duck near the bridge, show me the middle hill.

Understandably, Daisy can't get her head round this last question and so scores 4 out of 5.

After four more painful 'River Scenes' the instructions continue:

"… Inform patient you are now going to attempt something a little different. Ask him… (There is no 'her' included here, maybe after a few meetings, discussions and pilot schemes a politically approved 'her' will be included in these instructions)

To name as many animals as he can think of in 1 minute.

The helpful rubric sadly notes,

If patient appears doubtful, explain that you want the names of any kind of animal, wild or domestic.

Daisy churns out all the names of animals on the farm and their baby versions, but still only gets 6/10. Daisy who has seen pigs born and cows milked and pigs slaughtered, and who probably knows more about animals and different breeds than you and me. The Frenchay/Aphasia Screening sheet then reverts relentlessly once more to the 'River Scene'.

Now Daisy has given up. "Wasn't looking " is noted. She scores zero and is referred for Speech & Language Therapy. The next page perplexedly notes, "Normally very chatty and articulate and wide vocabulary. Very drowsy but conversational about her tortoiseshell cat Pearl."

Daisy has not had a speech-impairing right-side stroke.

Money Assessments are abandoned when Daisy fails to identify 31p. Reported as feeling "muddled", and when asked if she would like to stop, she replies simply, "Yes" and asks for a cup of tea instead. She would be happy to complete the assessment tomorrow because now she is drinking her tea and watching a film. The assessment is never completed.

The Visual Attention Assessment is not completed either: "Difficulties likely due to inattention?"

A carotid endarterectomy (a procedure to treat artery disease and reduce the risk of another stroke) was not performed. There is no indication why, when it was noted to be considered, this was then withdrawn.

A week after admission, a note is left for the dieticians.

MUST (Malnutrition Universal Screening Tool) score 3 (High Risk). Weight dropped from 48kg to 37kg. Food chart commenced. Build up milkshakes offered between meals.

In Bournemouth Hospital, on her admission on September 22nd, they asked me her weight. Daisy didn't live with me, and I didn't know her weight exactly, but I took a quick guess, thinking of my own weight and taking some kilos off, and I went for 48. 'History from mother' is not, this time, written beside this number. One day, walking early into the ward, I see Daisy is finishing a powdered supplement breakfast. (She liked this.) She is being fed up. They had weighed her. Thirty-seven kgs, a loss of 10 kgs in a few days. (No-one ever wanted to, or did, delete my guess of 48kgs, which remains on her notes).

Did no-one stop to consider the sums? In one week, a loss of 11 kilograms or 25 pounds. Having a stroke might have to be the most amazing diet plan ever devised.

Daisy is also anaemic, so anaemic she may require a blood transfusion.

ROYAL BOURNEMOUTH HOSPITAL
OCTOBER 1, 2012
STUCK IN HOSPITAL

Ten days after the stroke, Daisy is reported as "not her usual self as previously very chatty." Daisy, used to pottering about, now needs help to even turn over in bed. Lying in wet sheets, bored. How to occupy the long days now, between what? Sometimes, without warning, a therapist appears. The therapist objects to her staying overnight back in her flat and lists reasons, one of which was that the bed she would sleep in did not have cot sides. Yet somehow, many times, in the hospital, stroke patients, determined to somehow move for themselves, are found lying tumbled on the floor. Staff reaction is to be cross and accusatory (and write this in notes).

Forty years previously, we didn't know the questions to ask, but the care and attention Daisy received had been progressive, questioning and thoughtful. There was a willingness to explore all possible avenues.

Twenty years ago, Daisy had benefitted from the opportunity for two smart consultants to put their cutting-edge research into treatment and prone positioning of patients in ICU with ARDS.

Forty years on, we find the post stroke treatment dull, almost casual, unhelpful and poorly coordinated. The numerous 'Pathways' and protocols blunt the ability to respond to individuals. The patient clunks through the system, but too many do not fit and fall by the wayside. Daisy's irregular physiotherapy (the records show that in a sixty-four-day hospital stay she had only eleven physio sessions, including group sessions, after initial assessment, which itself was not completed "as drowsy".) The failures in communication and the thoughtless application of rules is our depressing legacy.

On discharge, Daisy has no physiotherapy, none at all. We seek out private physiotherapy which still continues. It later emerges that the NHS physiotherapy referral was not properly followed up. Too late for Daisy. Is Daisy's luck exhausted now?

But Daisy remains impossibly cheery (mostly). Sort of lucky Daisy again. Lucky not to lose her sight after the brain stem tumour removal, lucky not to die when unable to get any air into her lung with the fat embolism, lucky not to lose her speech or her verve after the stroke.

NOVEMBER 16, 2012

Graduating from a walk out of hospital grounds to the Tesco, or those walks in the hospital grounds (we peered into many strange buildings on the site, usually finding our way back past the bike sheds where off duty staff stood outside, smoking), almost two months later Daisy finally leaves hospital for a whole day. We drive back to her flat. There is Pearl, rescue cat Pearl, bought to keep down the mice (not to bring in half mangled baby birds), green eyes, black pupils, waiting. Pearl sizes up the wheelchair. We just sit together that day, Daisy, Pearl and me, on the sofa, have lots of cups of tea....and drive back to hospital for the night to find that, for the seventh time since admission, she has been moved bed again.

Next day, Daisy completes a Mood Rating Scale chart, "I feel...", which shows seven round faces in a row ranging from an open-mouthed laughing face, to one of utter despair. Pre-emoji days. Daisy has circled the scowling face next to last in which two hands are clutching the head in desperation. Beside this have been written Daisy's comments. "I feel cross that I have been moved" and "I can't sleep because of the noise of the bins." This was the pedal bin in the corner of the ward, which was banged open and shut almost every time someone passed it. The bins were never moved.

In stroke units, patients who recover movement within the allotted time trundle off to physio sessions (irregularly). Those who can't move are left in bed until there is someone available to help them. But they are in bed for many hours, described as 'prolonged bed rest'. So it is common practice to give Dalteparin injections, nightly. Dalteparin is used to prevent blood clots (deep vein thrombosis (DVT) which can lead to blood clots in the lung.) A DVT can occur in people who are bed-ridden. A risk assessment should be completed. In Daisy's case the risk assessment form was uncompleted, but she was still 'offered' the nightly torture, and when I gave up trying to persuade her, was duly recorded as 'patient refused'.

Dalteparin is given as an injection inserted under the skin of the stomach. It bruises the skin, making deep dark purple bruises, and Daisy objected. Perhaps her objection was to blunt needles, less experienced staff (it makes a difference) or to the creeping stain across her stomach. Daisy was not bed-ridden. She was never lying in bed all day. We wrapped her up in coats and blankets and duvets and shawls and, lying helpless in a sloping wheelchair, wheeled her to the hospital canteen for a second breakfast, chose the usual egg, bacon, toast, and drank too much coffee. (I was not able to drink coffee again for two years afterwards, without feeling sick.) We pushed her endlessly, round a lake in the hospital grounds or escaped the hospital confines across the road to a Tesco store where we drank more tasteless coffee and where we began to learn about the world of disabled toilets.

Let's go back.

POOLE HOSPITAL
DECEMBER 23 1996

Daisy leaves hospital, discharged, two days before Christmas. She looks composed and well. Everything; the voice activated furry parrot that had hung above her bed in ICU, the toys and books and CDs, the earphones and bags of gifts and cards and the hospital crutches, are piled into the car. She is tucked up in the back, wrapped in a cream cellular hospital blanket, in her gold Doc Martens boots and wearing a flowered headband. William puts his head on her lap. The best long drive home. The best Christmas ever. Safe. The pin in the leg is eventually removed eighteen months later. Small, neat scars are just visible on ankle and knee. The leg itself is perfectly straight again. But now in 2021, that leg will never, ever again, really work anymore.

Daisy's first real shoes were bright red, shiny, little trendy boots. We had to hunt the streets of downtown Tehran to find the smallest size. Four decades on, I hunt still for shoes. This time for shoes that can accommodate a left leg splint, shoes that need to be pushed and wriggled over the rainbow-decorated splint that keeps her post-stroke dead leg steady. That leg, with an almost invisible neat scar on the knee and on the ankle, a leg, which even before the stroke, had already been broken and had been put back and held together with a long slim pin.

DAISY'S FLAT, WEST MOORS, DORSET.
NOVEMBER 22, 2012

Daisy is wheeled out of Bournemouth Hospital, and waits, alone, wrapped up in coats and blankets against the dull and cold November day, while I go to retrieve the car. Escape once again. Escape for good. Her social worker is there as we leave. We drive back to her annexe flat, a drive I have been making for the last month.

At the flat, we meet the agency manager and the carer who will be looking after Daisy, who now needs 24/7 care (because she cannot walk unaided). The carer is young and direct. This is the first time she has seen Daisy. She knows nothing at all about her. Nobody knows anything about anything. The agency have not accepted the hospital's offer of a physio briefing. A hospital bed, with a stiff purple plastic mattress and clanking side bars, has been installed in her bedroom. It is a bleak homecoming. Stroke is the word. At a stroke, the life you have disappears. At a stroke, you must permit others to penetrate every minute of your day and night, and every minute part of your life. A brutal moment.

Swallowing my fear, I leave Daisy and return to Brighton. Two years of agency care are to follow. The agency, appointed by Social Services, are responsible for 20 hours care of each 24-hour day. The farm continues to provide 4/5 hours support, as they did before Daisy had her stroke.

In order to allow Daisy to return to her cat, her annexe flat, her former life (sort of), we need to resist letting Daisy be dumped in a residential home, and struggle to obtain a package that will allow her to resume 'normal' life. The ins and out of the systems, rules, regulations are completely unknown to me. However, just as every time before, the instinct is to carry on, to keep 'normal'. In reality, one wants to sit down and weep and weep and weep.

The agency chosen does their best. They really do. Educated Polish or Spanish girls appear and disappear. Older, wise English women employed by the agency speak up about the iniquities of the care system and the absurd pay rates, but are eventually defeated and, sadly, give up and leave. Most carers cope brilliantly, but some find Daisy's, direct approach to life a bit disconcerting. Daisy herself must now submit to many, many indignities and has become a very vulnerable young woman.

The agency boss promises to assemble a team to look after Daisy. A 'team' never ever materializes. In two years, Daisy had more than twenty different carers. One, unable to cope with a day when Daisy seems to be in extreme pain, just finds it easier gets her admitted to hospital but does not even stay with her. (It turned out that Daisy had a painful kidney infection.) Sam once again speeds down to visit her and is not admitted to the acute ward, as it is 'not visiting hours'. Olivia, a carer who has looked after Daisy, has a son who is a nurse at the hospital. Roundly and firmly, Olivia makes sure Sam is admitted to see Daisy. Daisy takes it in her stride. The rest of us are less sanguine.

Daisy's day is now crudely chopped up and determined by agency shifts. From 2pm to 10am the next morning it is the agency carer. From 10am to 2pm each day, the Farm looks after Daisy. Nobody has been trained or advised or helped how to look after Daisy. How to help her get up out of her chair, how to stand, how to turn her, how to sit, how to get her dressed (without wrenching the dead shoulder) or to wash her, how to help her eat food, with one hand, from a slippery plate (it took us scuffling in drawers in Bournemouth Hospital to find that there are, in fact, plate guards and specially designed left or right-handed cutlery; this was not provided routinely for stroke patients), how to turn her in bed, how to call for help, to get a cup of tea, to reach that biscuit, to pick up something from the floor, to scratch an itch, how to....how ...to be. Each person does it a little differently. Daisy is grabbed and pushed and pulled and tugged and touched. It would drive a saint mad. But almost like Tim in his extreme illness, Daisy becomes, somehow, most of the time, (a little) less stroppy.

Now Daisy begins a second life of tests and assessments; blood tests, eye tests, ear syringing. anaemia testing, medication reviews, assessments for alterations to the bathroom and later for a powered wheelchair. Along with other criteria, 'clients' need to show they can first control a powered chair in their home before they can use it outside. Daisy, some years before, had sat on Tim's lap in the car having a go at driving; she managed to demolish the wooden fence of the garden of our house in the country before Tim was able to stop the car. (During this incident, Sam, who had also been in the car, had wisely decided to abandon ship, and jumped out of the car before the crash.) Daisy sets off in 'Zippy' in her small flat reaches the hall wall and is stuck. Reversing, beeping, the shiny red chair chips the wall. The occupational therapists swallow hard. A five- or seven-point turn gets her to the kitchen arca. The day's trial ends. Soon, a final assessment will take place to see how Daisy is getting on. She's actually getting on quite well, in a Daisy sort of way. In a phone call she tells me she went out in Zippy.

"What do you mean 'out'?"

Daisy had taken matters into her own hands and gone out, although it was only just up the road and back.

dis = negative
disabled = unable to use a limb or limbs.

We never really considered what life was like for Daisy all those years ago; we just fought, and fought, and, in a way, resisted disability and tried to carry on as normal.

But as an adult, it is all very different, or is it, for Daisy?

A wheelchair sends a very strong signal and attitudes already adjust. But everywhere is different. Once, in Spain, in a large supermarket, I eventually located the person who had the key for the 'disabled' loo. It took some searching. Then we found our way down a crammed narrow corridor, clearing our way through boxes and, eventually, into the dark unlit loo. For once, I felt exasperated, and as I handed the key back, said I thought it was all rather *complicado*. The woman looked at me seriously and explained maybe that was because there weren't many disabled people in Spain.

However, although disabled people are less visible in Spain, we always encounter immense kindness. We brave the Carrefour shopping centre. It seems to me the only route back to the car park is down the moving escalator. (It had been a bit of a struggle to stop the wheelchair sliding backwards on the way up). Now we have loaded bags of shopping too. We set off. I assume the wheelchair will behave as a supermarket trolley and the wheels will lock. They don't. The speed rapidly gathers. I cling on as a man in office shirt and tie flings down his briefcase and vaults over the railings to help slow the runaway chair with Daisy in it. Shouting. People appear from below from their parked cars and swarm up the down escalator, forming a human barrier. My Spanish for both house building (we were in the process of reforming our little house) and giving thanks (many religious phrases) is pretty good.

In our small Spanish town, the disabled parking space (one) is routinely ignored. Pavements disappear abruptly and steep streets are too difficult to negotiate. Orange trees block the path. When we try to find a different route, winding through delightful narrow alleyways, we are then maddeningly confronted by a long flight of steps or a precipitous street. Foiled.

A new, portable powered wheelchair gives Daisy a new lease of life - she can turn and look, she can move where she wants. But her face says sad sometimes as the reality of this life pushes into her head.

We will go on. I treasure her existence, but I am sad too.

There is no real end to Daisy's story, but if you ask me what happened, this is what happened, all those years ago, and in those twenty-seven days in November.

Appendix

1971	1974	1995	2012	2021
Born	2years 7 months old	25 years old	41 years old	50 years old
	Brain tumour	Broken leg	Stroke	Alive to tell my story

A FEW CHEMICAL COCKTAILS: Daisy's drugs.

1974. THE BRAIN TUMOUR. A complete record of these drugs given is unknown as NHS Trust has a policy where records are not kept after 7 years.

Cobalt 60, a synthetic radioactive isotope produced artificially in nuclear reactors.

Cytosar, approved for use in 1969, a chemotherapy medication

Somatonorm, a synthetic human growth hormone, only approved in the US in 1985

Vincristine, approved in 1961, a chemotherapy medication

Ketamine, for starting and maintaining anaesthesia, approved for use in US in 1970

1997. THE BROKEN LEG

Medazepan, a sedative

Alfentimil , diamorphine - for pain

Dopemine, a cardiac stimulator 'flogger'

Dopexamine, a stimulant for heart failure in critically ill patients

Injections of Decapeptyl, a hormone treatment used alongside surgery or radiotherapy

Adrenaline, increases blood pressure, heart rate and cardiac output. An emergency heart stimulant
Insulin, controls blood sugar
Heperin, thins blood
Glyceryl trinitrate, takes strain off heart
Ventolin, a bronchial dilator
Fresubin, a tube feed nutritional drink
Cefotaxime, a broad-spectrum antibiotic
Ceftazadime, an antibiotic
Gentamicime, an antibiotic
Nystatin, anti-fungal
Furosemide, a diuretic
Temazepan, a relaxant
Paracetamol
Tricolfos, an oral sedative syrup
Norcuron, skeletal muscle relaxant used during mechanical ventilation
Sucralfate, to prevent duodenal ulcers

IN BETWEEN.
Amlodipine, for high blood pressure
Fluoxetine, to regulate mood
Metfomin, for Diabetes Type 2
Tegretol, for epilepsy
Tresiba, Insulin for Diabetes

2013 - CURRENT   THE STROKE
Clopidogrel, reduces risk of heart disease and stroke
Ferrous sulphate, treats iron deficiency anaemia
Metformin, a first-line medication for diabetes
Omeprazole, reduces stomach acid
Ramipril, treats high blood pressure
Simvastatin, lipid (fatty acid) lowering medication
Sitagliptin, anti-diabetic medication

Lansoprazole, reduces stomach acid
Amlopodine, treats high blood pressure
Dalteparin, a blood thinner

Acknowledgements

Dr Ken Power and Dr Barry Newman at Poole Hospital, 1996

Mr John Currie at Barts, 1974

Dr Anthony Hopkins & Liz

Becky (Dr Jarvis)

Geoffrey Walker and all staff in ICU, Poole, 1996

Many, many people have helped and supported us and I am so grateful. The people here have a special significance. Linda John & Clare, Teacher Libby Lodh and headmaster Trevor Jeavons, Pat Simcox, Rachel McFarlane, Evelyn Davies, Ann Thomson, Chris Austin, Hugh & Vanessa Arbuthnott, Hilary & Graham Laurie, Jane & Peter Fiddick & Harriet & Jonathan Turley, Nassrin & Abbas, Subi Swift & Amy, The Flacks, Marcus & Kate Konig Amy & Jenny, Tim & Georgina Woodward, Julia Midgely. Carers: Mhairi, Bronwyn, Olivia, Barbara, Cheryl, Michelle, Turkmen, Loren, Harriet, Louise, Miriam, Sula, Shipa. Physios: Holly, Nikki.

Sue Wells (& Martin) who didn't give up encouraging me to get this done. Emma Timpany, invaluable help.

Terri Patrick, Kay & Bernie Byrne, Jane & Oss, Sue & Terry Eliott, Gill, Jeff & the girls, Adelene & Joe, Sarah & Jake & Ken, Kevin, Carl & MacKenzie, Lesley, Brenda, Linda, Patricia, Sarah (riding), Bienvenido.

Endnotes

[i] Ataxic gait – a person's unsteady staggering movement which may result from abnormalities in different parts of the nervous system including the central nervous system (brain and spinal cord).

[ii] Dr. Anthony Hopkins, neurologist, our friend, was born in Poole, Dorset. When he died suddenly and unexpectedly, too young, in 1997, Daisy would be once again in hospital, in Poole.

[iii] Farlex Partner Medical Dictionary

[iv] Mosby's Medical Dictionary 2009

[v] Tobey J MacDonald MD

[vi] American Brain Tumor Association

[vii] The Mayo Clinic notes on Grand Mal seizures

[viii] American Lung Association Fact Sheet

[ix] Extracted from CSI Medicine

[x] Extract from Abstract by Jacqui Beltz and Heather Butler, Second Year Medicine, University of Tasmania

[xi] NeurosurgFocus 36; Aatman M Shah BC, Henry Jung MD, Stephen Skirboll MD, Stanford University California.

[xii] Jan Powers PhD, CCRN, CCNS, CNRN, FCCM   2011

[xiii] Historical Perspectives in Cardiology, A Viewpoint, Kanu Chatterjee, MB, FRCP (Lond.) FRCP (Edin.)

[xiv] extracted from Marcus E Raichle, Behind the scenes of functional brain imaging: A historical and physiological perspective. The National Academy of Sciences in the USA, February 3, 1998, vol 95, no.3.

[xv] Ramathan Ramprasad and Mukul Chandra Kapor, Journal of Anesthesiology Clinical Pharmacology 2012.

[xvi] Steven B Greenberg, MD Jeffrey Vender, MD, MBA, FCCP, FCCM, The Use of Neuromuscular Blocking Agents in the ICU, Critical Care Medicine 2013. Medscape, Spain.

[xvii] Geoffrey Walker, now Matron for Modern Medicine, Cardiology and Specialist Services, at Poole Hospital. Geoffrey Walker, OBE. JP. Geoffrey Walker, Nurse of the Year 2013, nominated by his colleagues. Geoffrey was the staff nurse in ICU at Poole Hospital in 1996 when Daisy was a patient there.

[xviii] Brian Moylan. online. Drugs 30/01/12

[xix] Pressure support mechanical ventilation was first introduced in 1982.

[xx] A History of Cancer Chemotherapy 2008 68; 8643, Vincent T, DeVita Jnr, and Edward Chu

Printed in Great Britain
by Amazon